AVIATION MEDICINE

AVIATION MEDICINE

Richard M Harding, BSc, MB, BS, PhD, DAvMed,
AFOM, MRAeS
*Wing commander, RAF Institute of Aviation Medicine,
Farnborough, Hampshire*

F John Mills, MB, BCh, DAvMed, Dip Pharm Med, PhD
*Senior vice president, Europe, Corning Pharmaceutical Services;
lately squadron leader, RAF Institute of Aviation Medicine,
Farnborough, Hampshire*

with contributions from

Roger Green, BSc
*Principal psychologist, Army Personnel Research Establishment,
Farnborough, Hampshire*

P J C Chapman, MB, DPH
*Lately chief medical officer, British Caledonian Airways Ltd,
Crawley, West Sussex*

and

Terence E Martin, BSc, MB, BS, DRCOG,
Dip IMC RCS(Ed), DAvMed, MRAeS
*Research medical officer, RAF Institute of Aviation Medicine,
Farnborough, Hampshire; lately trauma registrar, Helicopter
Emergency Medical Service, Royal London Hospital*

Published by the BMJ Publishing Group
Tavistock Square, London WC1H 9JR

First edition 1983
Second impression (with corrections) 1985
Second edition November 1988
Second impression 1991
Third edition 1993

British Library Cataloguing in Publication Data

A catalogue record for this book is available from the British Library.
ISBN 0–7279–0814–6

Typeset, printed and bound in Great Britain by
Latimer Trend & Company Ltd, Plymouth

Acknowledgments

Our thanks are due to many colleagues who helped in the preparation of the original series of articles. In particular, we are indebted to air vice marshal P Howard, group captain D Glaister, surgeon commander AP Steele-Perkins, Dr AJ Benson, Dr DH Brennan, Mr RG Green, Dr AJF Macmillan, Barbara Stone, and Dr JL Wheale, RAF Institute of Aviation Medicine; Dr Roger L Green and Dr FS Preston, British Airways Medical Service; Dr Peter Chapman, British Caledonian Medical Service; Dr G Bennett, Civil Aviation Authority; the Medical Protection Society; and Mr St John Chester, barrister at law.

In addition, it is a pleasure to acknowledge the advice of Doctors RB MacLaren and Sandra Mooney of the British Airways Medical Service, Dr RA Pearson of the Civil Aviation Authority, and Dr M Bagshaw during the preparation of the second edition.

For their generous help and advice during the preparation of the third edition, our grateful thanks are due once again to Dr Sandra Mooney and Dr M Bagshaw of the British Airways Health Services, and to Dr RA Pearson of the Civil Aviation Authority. It is also a pleasure to acknowledge the assistance of Dr JRR Stott and Lt Col RW Weien US Army, of the RAF Institute of Aviation Medicine.

Contents

Introduction

I find the great thing in this world is not so much where we stand as in what direction we are moving.

Oliver Wendell Holmes (1809–1894)

Most of the chapters in this book were originally published in the *British Medical Journal* in the summer of 1983. In a valediction for the 20 week series[1] we noted that critics of such an extensive review of aviation medicine might have been forgiven for thinking that the journal had succumbed to the national euphoria for marathons while upholding the other great British virtue of supporting minority interests. In reality, aviation medicine has made a major and vital contribution to the development of the aeronautical and space industries, which in turn have had as great an impact on our lives as any of the other remarkable examples of twentieth century technological achievement.

In the time taken by the athlete to run a marathon it is possible for the healthy and the infirm alike to travel thousands of miles by air. In chapters 1 and 3 we have highlighted the medical problems that could arise for passengers and patients in the abnormal environment of flight. In particular we have examined the need for improvement and standardisation of emergency medical facilities aboard aircraft, and emphasised the legal, ergonomic, and clinical problems which complicate the treatment of inflight medical emergencies. In 1983, in the hope of stimulating debate, we made several recommendations for consideration by the medical profession, the airlines, and government. Many pertinent comments were forthcoming from our peers, but a constructive response from organisations such as the International Air Transport Association and the International Civil Aviation Organization was not prompt. In 1981, the annual representative meeting of the British Medical Association had declined an opportunity to debate some of the questions that we raised, and a further opportunity was offered at the 1983 meeting but was again ignored. The *BMJ* did, however, commission and publish a paper by Dr Peter Chapman on the legal aspects of medical treatment in the air (chapter 2).

1

In 1984, the British Medical Association established a working party to consider the problems of aeromedical transportation of the sick and injured. Other working parties have been established more recently, and this is a reflection of the increasing importance this topic now has. We too have moved with the times, and a new chapter by Dr Terence Martin on the transport of patients by air is a welcome addition to this work (chapter 4). Unfortunately, the management of illnesses occurring during scheduled flights is not often within the remit of such working groups, but many airlines have taken it upon themselves to rationalise and improve the medical and first aid kits provided on board their aircraft—for example, the updated kits used throughout the British Airways fleet, and the semi-automatic defibrillators now carried on long haul Qantas flights—and to improve the training provided for their staff, often to paramedical standards (chapter 1).

The commercial airlines have matched their technological progress with a remarkable safety record, but there is still room for improvement and this is particularly so in relation to accident survivability. In the 10 years since we first wrote on this subject it is pleasing to note—although sadly at some cost in human tragedy—that many of the problems described in 1983 have been or are being actively addressed. Lives are still lost, however, because the aviation industry and its regulators have not yet overcome the limitations imposed by international bureaucracy and internal resistance to the introduction of, for example, rearward facing seats and more structurally sound materials for cabin furnishings. Even as the original papers were written, people died as a result of a fire on board an Air Canada DC9: all 23 deaths occurred after landing and were due to toxic fumes. The year 1985 was particularly bad for aircraft accidents, including as it did several fatal events on the ground either after landing or on takeoff. In the latter group, most notably for the United Kingdom, was the Boeing 737 disaster at Manchester airport. As described in chapter 9, this accident, and others like it, prompted the aviation authorities to look more closely at the construction of cabin furniture, at the installation of fire warning and fire fighting equipment, and at the possible provision of improved methods for ensuring personal survival—for example, smokehoods for crew and passenger use, floor level lighting, and audio tone devices to guide passengers to exits. However, in 1989 the Kegworth disaster claimed 47 lives when another Boeing 737 crashlanded on the M1 motorway. Fire was not a crucial factor in this accident, but the integrity of cabin furnishings and seats was. And so it goes on: although the national aviation authorities are undoubtedly addressing many of these safety issues[2] it is sometimes difficult to understand why, in the face of so much evidence, improvements take quite as long as they do.

Emergency considerations are, thankfully, a relatively minor part of the day-to-day operation of commercial airlines. Of far greater importance to farepaying passengers are matters of aircraft catering, sanitation, cleanliness, and cabin air quality. Not quite so obvious, but equally important, is disease control; including, of course, the status of those infected with human immunodeficiency virus (HIV). Transmeridian travel and jet lag affect passengers and crew alike but, for the latter, aircrew scheduling which accommodates medical and commercial needs is particularly germane. These topics are dealt with in chapters 3 and 9. The recent plea by doctors from the Public Health Laboratory Service for wider recognition of Travel Medicine as a medical specialty was of directly related interest;[3] an aim which we wholeheartedly endorse.

From a medical standpoint, flight safety has long centred upon the fitness of the crew, with especial emphasis being placed on detection of cardiovascular disease. This approach underlined the limitations of predictive testing rather than provided a solution to the problems; and so it is gratifying to recognise the important contributions made in this area by the 1982 and 1987 United Kingdom Workshops in Aviation Cardiology, and by the First European Workshop in 1991. These successful ventures were initiated by British cardiologists with a particular interest in their specialty as it relates to aircrew licensing, and the guidelines produced are discussed in chapter 10, along with a consideration of other important aspects of crew fitness including respiratory and endocrine disorders, infection with HIV, self-medication, and the use of alcohol by aircrew.

For obvious reasons psychiatric disorders in aircrew are also sought actively, but it is in relation to normal psychological function and its limitations that perhaps the greatest inroads into improved flight safety can now be made (chapter 8). Although this need has long been recognised by the Civil Aviation Authority, which has given, and continues to give, substantial financial support to research in this connection, a great deal remains to be learnt about human factors, and it is here that future research must be concentrated.

As described in chapters 5, 6, and 7, however, the hard learned physiology of exposure to altitude, increased acceleration, and of the effects of flight on the special senses, must never be forgotten or ignored. Thus, hypoxia, hyperventilation, decompression illness and barotrauma are ever present, if remote, risks in modern civil and military aviation; while the agility of the next generation of fighter aircraft will be such that the acceleration physiologist–physician will be faced with problems for some time to come. Spatial disorientation and loss of situational awareness claim many lives each year; and statistics suggest that there has been little improvement over the past two decades, so this is yet another area where greater study is needed.

Chapters 11 and 12 deal with less usual, but no less important, forms of flight. Those enjoying the increasingly popular world of sports flying seem at times to adopt a cavalier attitude reminiscent of the early aviators. Such an approach is unacceptable for the 1990s and it behoves both the governing authorities and the medical practitioners concerned with aviation to ensure that regulation and education are appropriate to our present understanding of aviation medicine. The important world of rotary wing flying also deserves to shed its cinderella image: for too long the safety features of helicopter design have been subservient to the needs of cost effectiveness. The solutions to many design failings are well established and, it is pleasing to note, are now being reflected on the drawing boards of helicopter manufacturers.

Two major advances were made in the history of aviation during the 1960s: the development of supersonic transport aircraft and man's conquest of space. These special forms of flight present medical problems of considerable complexity, and their successful solution serves to emphasise that aviation medicine is in the forefront of the practice of preventive medicine. The development of supersonic transport provided medical advisers with a fascinating array of problems, including the effects of ionising radiation, ozone and kinetic heating: in fact, fears were largely unfounded and the high speed commuter can now travel safely beyond the speed of sound. Space travel has also required a vast physiological and medical input to solve its human problems. Problems of spacecraft accelerations, microgravity, and life support systems are just a few of the hurdles which had to be overcome: without the clear contributions of the world's life scientists there is no doubt that humans would still be firmly attached to earth. Notwithstanding the setback caused by the loss of the space shuttle Challenger, the long term effects of space on the individual remains an active field with the prospect of space laboratories, space stations, space settlements, and deep space exploration requiring a continual and continued research effort.

Aviation or aerospace medicine, then, has been and remains an exciting, growing, challenging, and adventurous specialty which touches all our lives: we are grateful to have been given the opportunity to share it with a wider audience.

Changes for the third edition

For the third edition of this book the opportunity has been taken to reorganise and revise many parts of the book, and to add new material; over 140 new references have been cited. The sections on jet lag, motion sickness, inflight crew incapacitation, cardiovascular fitness of aircrew, alcohol use by aircrew, and ionising radiation have been extensively updated while new sections on cabin air quality, fire and impact protection in civil aircraft, the regulation of air safety and aircrew licensing, HIV infection in aircrew, and the female pilot have been added. The most obvious change is the inclusion of a chapter on aeromedical transport, an area of endeavour which has grown enormously over the past decade.

1 Mills FJ, Harding RM. Aviation medicine—a valediction. *BMJ* 1983; **287:** 543.
2 Edgington K. Making air crashes more survivable (letter). *BMJ* 1992; **305:** 119.
3 Porter JDH, Stanwell–Smith R, Lea G. Travelling hopefully, returning ill (editorial). *BMJ* 1992; **304:** 1323–4.

Bibliography

For those who wish to read further about aviation medicine two definitive textbooks are recommended, one from the United Kingdom and the other from the United States. They are:

Ernsting J, King PF, eds. *Aviation medicine*, 2nd edn. London: Butterworths, 1988.
de Hart RL, ed. *Fundamentals of aerospace medicine*. Philadelphia: Lea and Febiger, 1985.

Additional information on all aspects of the health of travellers, including mountain sickness, a subject about which aviation medicine specialists are frequently consulted, can be found in:

Dawood RM, ed. *Travellers' health*, 3rd edn. Oxford: Oxford University Press, 1992.

Other books of interest and relevance include:

Bagshaw M, Campbell RD. *Human performance and limitations in aviation*. Oxford: Blackwell Scientific, 1991.
Green RG, Muir H, James M, Gradwell DP, Green RL. *Human factors for pilots*. Aldershot: Avebury Technical, 1991.
Harding RM. *Survival in space—medical problems of manned spaceflight*. London: Routledge, 1989.
Hawkins FH. *Human factors in flight*, 2nd edn. Aldershot: Ashgate Publishing, 1993.
Nicogossian AE, Leach-Huntoon C, Pool SL, eds. *Space physiology and medicine*, 2nd edn. Philadelphia: Lea and Febiger, 1989.
Rayman RR. *Clinical aviation medicine*, 2nd edn. Philadelphia: Lea and Febiger, 1990.

The following journals regularly publish original articles, reviews, and items of general interest on aviation medicine and related topics:

Aviation, Space and Environmental Medicine. The journal of the Aerospace Medical Association (monthly).
Travel Medicine International (quarterly).
Flight International (weekly).
Aviation Week and Space Technology (weekly).

1
Medical emergencies in the air

But a Samaritan, as he journeyed, came to where he was; and when he saw him, he had compassion.[1]

Air France has estimated that for three of every four life threatening medical emergencies occurring during flight a doctor is a passenger on board the aircraft.[2] According to Air Canada the incidence may be as high as 90%[3] whereas internal surveys by other airlines mention lower figures (40–50%). Some of the doctors who have responded to requests for medical assistance during flight have been critical of the emergency medical facilities provided; others have been disturbed by the lack of diagnostic and therapeutic equipment aboard aircraft,[4-8] the apparent failure of airlines to screen passengers for their fitness to fly,[5] and the lack of gratitude expressed by the airline to the doctor who has responded unselfishly to the emergency.[8] In an American study of 42 doctors who had responded to a total of 62 incidents,[9] only one considered the medical equipment on board the aircraft to be adequate and just five received written thanks from the airline. In the United States, following pressure from groups such as the Public Citizen Health Research Group and the Aviation Consumer Action Project,[3] the Federal Aviation Administration has since August 1986 required United States airlines to carry expanded medical kits.[10] Furthermore, airlines are required to report on the use of such kits, by whom they were used, and with what outcome. Although as yet there is no standardised reporting procedure, the first year of the scheme saw 1016 inflight incidents notified; and physicians responded in 63%.[11]

The views expressed in this chapter are our own and do not necessarily reflect those of British Airways, the Civil Aviation Authority, or the Royal Air Force.

Incidence of medical emergencies

Some doctors appear to have an "ancient mariner" effect[4] while travelling by air and find themselves attending numerous inflight emergencies; others—probably the majority—have never been troubled. The few statistics on such instances come from reviews of flight attendant reports, analyses of the number of unscheduled landings made for medical reasons or the number of inflight deaths, and information actively solicited from doctors who have been concerned in such incidents. These figures have to be interpreted with care because many factors, such as the nature of the airline's operation and its willingness or otherwise to accept seriously ill patients for humanitarian reasons, may bias the results. For example, a domestic airline may have a lower incidence of inflight deaths than an international airline simply because an aircraft can be diverted to another airport more rapidly on an overland domestic flight than on an intercontinental transoceanic route.

A review was undertaken 10 years ago of all inflight accident and medical incident reports submitted by British Airways cabin staff during 1979–80, when over 17 million passengers were carried.[12] Of the 1063 accidents reported, only eight were considered to be "major" (three cases of fracture, two of concussion, one of laceration requiring sutures, one of dislocation, and one of loss of consciousness); there were eight deaths during flight. Half the accidents occurred to flight attendants, and so the chance of a passenger having a "major" accident was remarkably small (one in 4·25 million). Interestingly, the overall ratio of flight attendant to passenger accidents was 3·7:1, which reflects both the greater mobility of the first group within the aircraft and the importance of including the crew in all surveys. By contrast, only four of a total of 1328 medical incidents concerned the crew, so that the "attack rate" for passengers was about one in 13 000—the same figure as that quoted by Qantas[13] for passengers needing inflight care by doctors or nurses during 1977, although the corresponding figure for 1976 was one in 21 000. In passengers whose disability had been notified to British Airways before the flight the rate was one in 350—a finding similar to that of the Air France Medical Department.[14]

The ratio recorded by British Airways of incidents on intercontinental flights to those on European and domestic flights was nearly 4:1, but the incident rate for each flight cannot be calculated from the figures quoted,[12] and they cannot be compared with figures from other airlines because of differences in reporting procedures. The same can be said of the more recent Federal Aviation Administration inflight incident returns.[11] Crew reports need to be standardised to ensure that meaningful statistics are obtained. Nevertheless, a long flight may be expected to produce more medical problems because of the greater exposure to factors ranging from immobility and hypoxia to the effects of duty free alcohol. A reasonable prediction is that medical help will be sought (but not necessarily required) on one in 50 international flights on wide bodied aircraft.[13]

Causes

In 1982, the most common medical problems encountered by British Airways were associated with the central nervous system, followed by those due to stress and anxiety (16% of total), those affecting the cardiovascular system (15%), the alimentary system (12%), and the respiratory system (10%).[12] In an earlier study by the British Overseas Airways Corporation (BOAC) of 377 medical incidents,[15] 15 were due to angina, 24 to heart failure, one to cardiac arrest, 22 to dyspnoea, five to asthma, and one to pulmonary embolism. The most common incidents were neurological, with 55 episodes of fainting, six fits, and 33 of mental illness. More recently, in the period April 1990–March 1991, the aetiology of the 2139 inflight incidents on British Airways flights was much the same and included 429 vasovagal attacks (20%), 261 cases of diarrhoea (12%), 112 anxiety syndromes (5%), 96 asthmatic attacks (4·5%), 42 cases of angina (2%), and 26 heart attacks (1·2%): this represents an "attack rate" of about one in 11 500 passengers carried. In the following year this increased to about one in 10 000.

These studies, and others, were based on retrospective medical judgements, and information regarding the severity of medical problems was not always provided. Thus the severity can be gauged only indirectly from the need to make unscheduled landings, a decision which will be affected by the level of training of the cabin crew, in the absence of a doctor on board, and by the sophistication of the medical equipment carried. For example, between 1975 and 1979 Qantas made 16 unscheduled landings, of which ten were for chest pain or suspected myocardial infarction.[12] Between 1964 and 1968 American Airlines made an average of one unscheduled landing for every one million passengers carried,[16] which is high when compared with one in 8·5 million for British Airways in 1979–80,[12] undoubtedly because at that time American Airlines was flying only domestic routes. Rarely was a doctor on board at the time of these landings, so the diagnoses were based mainly on crew reports which sometimes lacked information. Although half of the landings were probably unnecessary, these instances have not been excluded from the analysis: heart attack (real or suspected) and chest pain accounted for 33 of the 105 reports, syncope for 21, and dyspnoea for 20. The 1016 returns made to the Federal Aviation Administration in the first year of its inflight incident reporting programme revealed a similar aetiological pattern: the usual presenting features were chest pain and syncopal episodes, nine people died in flight and a further three on the ground. At least 89 incidents led to diversion of the flight.[11]

Other recent surveys of inflight medical emergencies also support the view that the pattern of illness has changed little over the past two decades. In a 1-year (1985/86) prospective study of emergency calls to the Seattle-Tacoma International Airport, during which the airport saw 274 000 flights involving 14·4 million passengers, 190 people had inflight medical problems:[17] seven of these were on flights diverted for (probably unnecessary) medical reasons, and there were five cardiac arrests (including one inflight). The most common presentations were, however, the ubiquitous "others": nonspecific complaints, sleeplessness, and alcohol related problems. The most common specific complaint was gastrointestinal illness (pain, nausea, vomiting, and diarrhoea). Of considerable additional interest was the finding that passengers were twice as likely to be ill on the ground (before or after flight) than when airborne: such events accounted for another 564 cases. Another year-long survey carried out at Los Angeles International Airport during 1985/86 produced very similar findings: 260 passengers out of nearly 8·75 million arrivals had developed a medical problem in flight; once again the most common serious presentations were chest and abdominal pain, and loss of consciousness.[18] There was one fatality per 1·3 million passengers.

As these surveys indicate, cardiovascular disease is the most common cause of serious illness in passengers during flight, and this is confirmed by studies on deaths which have occurred from natural causes on board aircraft. In a wide ranging review of data from the 120 airlines in the International Air Transport Association, 577 passenger deaths inflight were recorded in the 8 years from 1977 to 1984.[19] Of these, most of which were of apparently previously healthy people, 66% were of middle-aged men. Fifty six per cent were sudden cardiac deaths, while cancers accounted for 8% and respiratory disease for 6%—a distribution of diagnoses similar to that seen in the 90 deaths reported in BOAC passengers from 1947 to 1967[15] and the 25 deaths reported more recently by Qantas.[13] During the year April 1991–March 1992, British Airways carried 25 million passengers. There were 2607 inflight incidents, and 23 diversions were made for medical reasons. Fourteen deaths occurred in flight, and in only two of these cases had the airline been informed beforehand of a medical problem.

Legal aspects of emergency care (see also chapter 2)

The provision of medical care by airlines during flight covers the selection of first aid kits, the training of flight attendants, and the allocation of adequate space for treatment. Certain legal considerations which apply to the airline and to itinerant doctors are of paramount importance.

All doctors should feel that they have a moral duty to help anyone in distress but in recent years there has been a trend for doctors not to declare themselves at accidents or emergencies for fear of subsequent litigation. Under the law practised in most British Commonwealth countries and in the United States there is no legal obligation to give aid to a stranger, but in most European countries it is a criminal offence not to render assistance. The legal onus to help will therefore depend on geography and possibly the nationality of the carrier. Geography may also be relevant should litigation ensue, because of medical insurance cover: for example, a British doctor on holiday in the United States will not be covered by his defence society for litigation arising in that country. The "wealth" of the airlines should perhaps be used to underwrite any damages[6] but the demise in the 1980s of Laker, Braniff, Spantax and other airlines has already been followed in the 1990s by that of Dan Air, Compass and Pan Am; and the undoubted financial problems of many of the major international carriers hardly support the notion that airlines in the 1990s are wealthy.

Of the 42 doctors in the American study who had responded to inflight incidents,[9] at least half were reluctant to answer requests for medical assistance, mainly because they were afraid that the problem would be outside their usual field of practice. This is understandable because inexperience may be no defence against allegations of negligence. For this reason airlines have to be cautious in their choice of equipment for first aid kits, lest it be beyond the expertise of the user. For example, endotracheal tubes should be provided for use by doctors,[4] but many doctors have not passed a tube for many years because of their specialisation. Under cramped, possibly turbulent, conditions it might be over optimistic to expect a successful intubation. Those who condemn this argument and can intubate with ease may still be subject to litigation because of their lack of experience in aviation medicine. For example, a rapid decompression to 10 668 m (35 000 ft) can produce endotracheal cuff pressures far above those known to cause tracheal damage. Would the doctor be aware of the need to correct the cuff pressure? Even when properly set for cruise altitude the cuff pressure can still fall below that required to prevent aspiration when the aircraft returns to sea level.[20]

Legal considerations also determine the choice of drugs for first aid kits. British operators might wish to make diamorphine available in an emergency kit for use by doctors, but their aircraft could then be impounded in the United States because they are carrying a drug which is prohibited even from controlled medical use in that country. The medical kit used by British Airways (see table 1.2 and below) contains several preparations which are otherwise only available on prescription; under certain well defined conditions these may be administered by a member of the cabin crew. Potential legal problems have been overcome by close cooperation with the Department of Health and other authorities, based on the firmest assurances that the use of these drugs will be correctly and dutifully recorded by crew attendants who have been trained in their use. Legal authority to prescribe and dispense has been given by the Department of Health and the Home Office, and is contained in instructions listed in the British Airways cabin crew manual.

Finally, to overcome these problems it has been suggested that doctors should take their medical bag along with them when travelling by air, being exempt from any excess baggage charges that may result.[7] This idea received support from the American Medical Association, which has even outlined a suitable list of medicines to be carried.[21] At present, however, this is impractical on all but domestic flights because most countries prohibit the import and export of medicines unless they are required for the person's own health or unless import/export has been previously approved. These regulations often include medicines other than controlled drugs, and doctors should be fully aware of their legal vulnerability in this area.

First aid equipment

All airlines are required by civil aviation regulations to carry first aid kits on all flights, the number per aircraft being dependent on the number of passenger seats. These so-called amenities kits are basic and contain bandages, surgical tape, antiseptics, et cetera, and usually a few proprietary medicines (most commonly analgesics, decongestants, and drugs for motion sickness). In addition, airlines are obliged to provide portable oxygen sets as well as emergency oxygen supplies. Some airlines, such as British Airways, now provide a more comprehensive kit for use by trained cabin crew, subject to the legal considerations already outlined. The first aid equipment and drugs contained in this kit are summarised in table 1.1. The controversial issue of whether a supplementary kit should also be provided for the sole use of doctors who might be on board has been discussed at length by the Medical Advisory Committee of the International Air Transport

TABLE 1.1—Contents of British Airways aircraft first aid kits

Hyoscine tablets	Finger dressings	Safety pins
Magnesium trisilicate tablets	Medium dressings	Disposable gloves
Paracetamol tablets	Large dressings	Biohazard bag
Merocets lozenges	Triangular bandage	Resusciade
Smelling salts	Bandages	
Vick inhaler	Micropore tape	
Savlon antiseptic cream	Bandaid	
Sulphacetamide eye drops	Steristrips	

In addition, for long haul routes

Paludrine tablets	Scissors
Insect repellant	First aid leaflet
Water testing set	Water supplies leaflet
Chloramine T tablets	

13

Association. Although this organisation aims to standardise medical equipment among its member airlines, decisions on the carriage and contents of kits for doctors only were until the mid 1980s the prerogative of the individual airline. The consensus is that such facilities should be available on board aircraft, and the Federal Aviation Administration has now made the carriage of such kits compulsory.[10] It was in anticipation of such statutory regulations that the British Airways M5 medical kit, which includes equipment and drugs for use by doctors, was introduced in 1988 to replace the A50 first aid kit (see table 1.2). Other airlines, such as Air France, Alitalia, Iberia, Lufthansa, and Sabena, had for some time already equipped their aircraft with kits for use *solely* by doctors. Qantas now carries semiautomatic defibrillators on all long haul flights: cabin staff are trained in their use as well as in cardiopulmonary resuscitation.

The provision of first aid kits is determined by four main factors.

(1) The level of expertise of the user must be assessed. Quite apart from legal considerations, the aircraft's environment may make the use of certain procedures difficult—for example, the monitoring of blood pressure with a stethoscope when there is noise and vibration.[22]

(2) The choice of drugs should not exceed the diagnostic capabilities of the attending doctor, which will in turn be limited by the level of equipment provided on board the aircaft. For example, certain antiarrhythmic drugs should be administered to patients only if an electrocardiograph is available. Furthermore, the nature of the medicines and their method of administration must be comprehensible to doctors of many nationalities.

(3) The kit must be secure from unauthorised use and theft. Airlines often find that articles of safety equipment, such as lifejackets and even loudhailers, are stolen by passengers; for this reason, spares are always carried. To guarantee security, modifications may have to be made to the aircraft's internal layout and the kits designed so as to ensure their accommodation in a range of different aircraft within a fleet. Procedures for checking contents and restocking of used and time expired items will have to be set out and enforced.

(4) Before the kit can be used, the crew must be able to identify the passenger as a medically qualified doctor, because unqualified people, for whatever motive, occasionally claim that they are

TABLE 1.2—Contents of British Airways M5 emergency medical case

Item	Quantity	Brief notes to user
In lid		
instruction handbook	1	
record form	1	
voyage report sheets	2	
"Used in flight" label	1	
pencil	1	
torch and batteries	1	Eye and throat examination
5-inch scissors	1	General use
safety pins (packet)	1	General use
British Airways seals	2	For security of locks
Sharpak needle/syringe holder	1	For disposal of used sharps and syringes
obstetric delivery pack (mucus extractor, cord clamps, scissors, forceps)	1	
aneroid sphygmomanometer*	1	
Litmann stethoscope*	1	
rubber tourniquet	1	To arrest bleeding
WOW cotton bandages	2	General use
triangular bandages	2	To support shoulder, hands, or limbs
wound dressings, small	2	
wound dressings, medium	2	
absorbent gauze squares (packet of five)	2	
Op-site wound dressing	2	Specialised wound covering
Mediswabs (packet of five strips)	2	Alcohol pad for skin sterilisation
Steristrips (packet of five strips)	6	Sterile wound closures
Savlon cream (15 g)	1	Antiseptic cream
Oral drugs		
buprenorphine hydrochloride (Temgesic) (packet of 10 tablets)	3	Treatment of pain
loperamide (Arret, Imodium) (packet of 12 capsules)	2	Treatment of diarrhoea
lorazepam (Ativan) (packet of 10 × 1 mg tablets)	1	Treatment of anxiety or insomnia

15

TABLE 1.2—Continued

Item	Quantity	Brief notes to user
isosorbide dinitrate (Isordil) (packet of two 5 mg sublingual tablets)	1	Treatment of angina—fast relief
Hypostop (three dose container)	1	Treatment of hypoglycaemia
salbutamol sulphate (Ventolin) (packet of six 2 mg tablets)	1	Treatment of mild asthmatic attack
salbutamol sulphate (Ventolin Rotacaps) (15 capsules plus rotahaler)	2	For prompt and continuing relief of acute asthmatic attack. Use with Ventolin tablets
In tray No 1*		
Injectable drugs		
nalbuphine hydrochloride (Nubain) (10 mg ml⁻¹ in preloaded syringe)	4	Treatment of acute pain, including that of myocardial infarction. Dose 10–30 mg IV, IM, or SC
adrenaline BP (1 ml ampoules of 1:1000)	2	Use to (a) arrest bleeding, (b) increase blood pressure and cardiac rate. Dose 0·2–0·5 ml SC
atropine (600 mg in 1 ml ampoules)	2	Cardiac conditions associated with vagal stimulation and bradycardia; antispasmodic action on smooth muscle. Dose 300–500 µg IM
aminophylline (250 mg in 10 ml ampoules)	2	Relieves bronchial spasm. Cardiac, pulmonary, or renal failure. Dose 250–500 mg IV
diazepam (Valium) (10 mg in 2 ml ampoules)	2	Acute anxiety state as sedative and in treatment of muscle spasm. Dose 5–10 mg IM or IV
digoxin (Lanoxin) (0–5 mg in 2 ml ampoules)	3	Congestive cardiac failure. Dose 0.1–0.3 mg IM or IV
promethazine hydrochloride (Phenergan) (25 mg in 2 ml ampoules)	2	Allergic conditions. Dose 25–50 mg deep IM
hyoscine butylbromide (Buscopan) (20 mg in 1 ml ampoules)	2	Gastrointestinal spasm, urinary tract spasm, renal stone. Dose 20 mg IM or IV
metoclopramide hydrochloride (Maxolon) (10 mg in 2 ml ampoules)	2	Nausea and vomiting due to gastrointestinal disorders. Dose max 0–5 mg kg⁻¹ IM or IV
dexamethasone (Decadron) (4 mg in 2 ml ampoules)	1	Emergency parenteral therapy. Intra-articular and soft tissue conditions. Dose up to 4 mg IV or IM
glucagon plus solvent (1 mg in 2 ml ampoules)	1	Acute hypoglycaemia. Dose 1 mg IV, IM, or SC

16

frusemide (Lasix) (20 mg in 2 ml ampoules)	2	Oedema, hypertension, renal insufficiency. Dose 20–50 mg single dose IM or slow IV
water for injection (2, 10, 20 ml ampoules)	2 each	General use

In tray No 2*

Injectable drugs

sodium bicarbonate (8·4%) (preloaded 50 ml syringe)	2	Metabolic acidosis in cardiac arrest. IV
isoprenaline hydrochloride (preloaded syringe, 0·2 mg in 10 ml)	2	Stimulant in cardiac arrest; bradycardia associated with heart block
calcium chloride (10%) (preloaded 10 ml syringe)	2	IV use
dextrose (50%) (preloaded 50 ml syringe)	1	Used in myocardial infarction in combination with calcium chloride. Slow IV
lignocaine hydrochloride (Xylocard) (100 mg in preloaded 5 ml syringe)	2	Ventricular dysrhythmias in connection with myocardial infarction. Dose 50–100 mg IV over 2 min.
metaraminol tartrate (Aramine) (10 mg in 1 ml ampoules)	1	Increases coronary blood flow and blood pressure. Dose 2–10 mg IM or SC
syntometrine		

In base*

urinary catheters	2
disposable syringes (2, 5, and 20 ml)	2 each
disposable needles (sizes 1, 12, 17, 21)	4 each
disposable scalpel	1
curved suture needles	6
Mersilene black polyester suture	3
Mediswabs (packet of five strips)	4

In lid flap

inflatable splint for arm	1
inflatable splint for leg	1

Aircraft emergency medical equipment

Oxygen
Ambu bag
Airways (three sizes)
Eye irrigator

*Not for cabin staff use.

17

physicians. Moreover, some practitioners may find it difficult to provide positive identification of their profession.

Doctors' kits

The main diagnostic additions to airline doctors' kits are a stethoscope, and a sphygmomanometer; the medicines carried vary but should include loperamide, glyceryl trinitrate, dexamethasone, a diuretic such as frusemide, adrenaline (epinephrine), diphenhydramine, nalbuphine, atropine, aminophylline, promethazine, hyoscine, metoclopramide, diazepam, and dextrose. Parenteral preparations have been recognised as particularly likely to "make a significant difference in the immediate treatment of several (relatively common) problems".[17] To overcome difficulties with identification, the generic name of each drug should be listed together with its major European and American trademarks. Information in English, German, Italian, Spanish, and French should also be available on each drug's usual dosage, the route of administration, and its indications and contraindications for use. The remaining contents of the doctor's kit are syringes, suture materials with appropriate sterile instruments, and airways; a laryngoscope and endotracheal tubes are not included. The complete kit is sealed and placed in a locked compartment, the key to which is held on the flight deck and released only with the captain's permission. Each time the kit is used a report is written by the chief steward and the doctor. Since 1975 Air France has extended the availability of its doctors' kits from its 747 fleet to all its long-haul aircraft and airbuses because they are "unquestionably useful to sick persons".[2] The British Airways *combined* cabin staff and doctors' medical kit, the comprehensive M5 (the contents of which are listed in table 1.2), is available on board all British Airways' aircraft in a single lockable holdall under the control of the captain. For more mundane or commonplace conditions the free access amenities kits will still be provided: the M1, which contains simple analgesics, nasal decongestants, throat lozenges, antiemetics, etc, on short haul, narrow bodied aircraft; and the larger M2, which also contains antimalarial tablets, insect repellant, and water testing equipment, for long haul, wide bodied aircraft (see table 1.1).

Although such equipment could decrease the number of costly diversions by stabilising emergencies on board,[23] there is as yet no clear statistical support for this: the Federal Aviation Administration's reporting scheme should, however, begin to redress this lack. In the meantime, the authors of the 1988 review of International Air Transport Association data concluded that their results "support the initiation of programmes to train cabin personnel in the skills of basic cardiopulmonary resuscitation and in the use of automatic external defibrillators".[19] Clearly, commercial considerations should not be used to persuade a doctor to continue treatment during flight to a level at which he or she might not be confident. For the same reasons oversophistication in medical kits may not be in the best interests of the patient. Nevertheless, there is a strong case for providing upgraded doctors' kits on transoceanic long haul flights, because an unscheduled landing may take up to 4 hours to effect. Under these conditions the airlines should perhaps take advantage of the improvements made in biotelemetry in the past 25 years;[24] thus a ground based cardiologist could relay an expert opinion on a dysrhythmia in a passenger who is thousands of miles away. Such a step would require considerable investment in equipment and a long, costly period of training in its use for at least one crew member in each aircraft. This exercise would presuppose that the attendant had also been trained to paramedic standards and so be allowed access to the drugs available in the medical bag because there can be no guarantee that a doctor will be on board. Apart from creating organisational and financial problems for the airline in ensuring that a trained and current paramedic is scheduled to be on every flight, this approach raises further legal and professional problems. Nevertheless, all those who have studied the matter report that current equipment and training are inadequate, and that there is an undoubted need for greater training for flight attendants.[17-26] Finally, if these shortcomings are addressed in full, extra space would have to be found to accommodate the additional equipment in a suitable treatment area.

Space for treatment

The economics of airline operations dictate that space on board aircraft is at a premium. On most aircraft a patient may lie flat only in the area surrounding emergency exits or, on larger aircraft, in galley areas or the first class compartment. Air Afrique and UTA (a large French independent airline) have installed a special medical compartment on their long-haul aircraft that provides room for resuscitation, isolation, and general medical assistance for seriously ill patients.[23] Under certain circumstances, particularly if cardiac arrest is suspected, movement to a treatment area would take too long to allow successful resuscitation. It may take up to 2 minutes for neighbouring passengers to recognise a cardiac arrest and another minute before a flight attendant arrives at the scene.[23] The mild hypoxia associated with a cabin altitude of several thousand feet means that time is even further limited and that resuscitation will have to be undertaken while the patient is in situ. Although the patient may be lain flat across two or three seats with the arm rests removed or in the up position (figure 1.1), removal of the patient to the aisle is probably the quickest and best method. To offset hypoxia, the rescuer performing ventilation should maintain a high Po_2 by breathing from an emergency 100% oxygen supply. All flight attendants should be well trained in cardiopulmonary resuscitation in view of the difficulties imposed by an aircraft environment.

Prevention of medical emergencies

As with any other branch of medicine, prevention of emergencies should be encouraged. Airlines do not generally make enough effort to screen passengers for their fitness to fly. Nevertheless, assuming that each airline has an advisory medical department, it is still not feasible for all passengers to be monitored; Heathrow airport alone handled 62 million passengers in 1992! A system is therefore needed that identifies those passengers at risk. The present reporting methods have deficiencies and, although the recommendations below could improve the situation, the very large numbers involved will still present problems. In 1987 British Airways Health Services reviewed applications from about 14 000 passengers with significant medical problems for their fitness to fly. Any increase in the number of cases will require further investment by the airlines in medical staff and facilities.

Recommendations

(1) All passenger carrying airlines should have a medical department in which at least one doctor has been trained in the specialty of aviation medicine. As long ago as 1981, because of economic pressures on the airlines, many medical departments were reduced in size or even eliminated. In 1982, in response to this, the Aerospace Medical Association resolved "That all airlines be

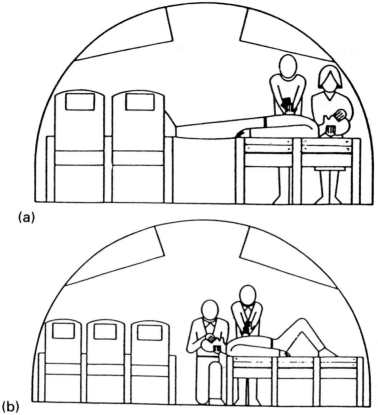

FIG 1.1—Cardiopulmonary resuscitation in an aircraft cabin using (a) two or (b) three seats abreast. The seat backs are not shown in the drawing so that the position of the resuscitators may be seen. An item such as a briefcase should be placed under the victim's chest to ensure effective cardiac massage. (Reproduced by permission of the editor of *Aviation, Space and Environmental Medicine.*)

encouraged to develop and maintain meaningful aerospace medical departments."[24] The present economic climate makes this even more unlikely.

(2) Passengers should be made more aware of the medical hazards of air travel. The present system of screening is unsatisfactory because it depends to a great extent on the medical alertness of the travel agent. Passengers who are ill are likely to have their tickets bought for them by a fit third party and it is unlikely that

medical problems will be picked up at this stage. Thus a warning to passengers about the health hazards of air travel should be printed on airline tickets in the same way that attention is given to the carriage of certain prohibited goods. To avoid adverse consumer reactions to those airlines which undertake such action voluntarily (and which may be assumed, incorrectly, by the passenger to be unsafe), all airlines should be obliged to comply with this recommendation.

(3) Doctors should be made aware of the medical problems that a patient may face when travelling by air. They are already encouraged to discuss medical problems with those airlines that have a medical department, and should make full use of this opportunity.

(4) The lack of statistics on medical incidents during flight needs to be remedied. The Aerospace Medical Association has already made some recommendations for improvement, but their success will depend on the standard of reporting. In particular, an internationally recognised protocol should be drawn up and adhered to by all airlines for the reporting of such incidents. The Federal Aviation Administration requirement is a step in the right direction.[10] The attendance of a doctor should be recorded for statistical purposes (to assess the severity of the complaint) and so that he or she may later be contacted and thanked by the airline.

(5) The standard of emergency medical facilities available on aircraft needs to be debated openly within the medical profession, based on the availability of information from the previous recommendation: there are signs that this too is being actively addressed.

(6) The legal implications of 'good samaritan' acts should be considered on a worldwide basis. Governments should examine the possibility of underwriting such actions on aircraft registered in their countries. Alternatively, the airlines should discuss the possibility of taking out comprehensive bulk insurance with agencies such as the medical defence societies.

(7) The airlines should consider training one crew member to paramedic standards, especially for long haul flights. Because in future aircraft may carry up to 800 passengers, the likelihood of a medical emergency arising is increased. The need for inflight treatment areas should also be thoroughly analysed. Such recommendations would also require legislation by national aviation authorities and probably cooperation between industries.[25] Here, too, there are indications that the airlines are acting on their own

initiative. In a worldwide analysis of flight attendant first aid training, 52 of 136 airlines questioned responded. Of the 50 which employed flight attendants, 96% provided annual first aid training, and 24% provided advanced training for senior staff. The study concluded that all airlines should provide 16 h of basic first aid training and testing (to include cardiopulmonary resuscitation) given by professional and appropriate teachers, with more extensive training being given to senior staff. Annual refresher courses were also recommended, along with the production of an airline first aid manual.[26]

1 St Luke, chap X, verse 33. *The Holy Bible* (revised standard version).
2 Pasquet J. Emergency medical kits aboard aircraft. *Aviat Space Environ Med* 1977; **49:** 882–5.
3 Anonymous. Suit seeks airline carriage of emergency medical gear. *Aviation Week and Space Technology* 1982; **117:** 41.
4 Rennie ID. Medical hazards of air travel. *BMJ* 1977; **ii:** 515.
5 Callaghan JG. Medical hazards of air travel. *BMJ* 1977; **i:** 1473–4.
6 McLaren HC. Medical hazards of air travel. *BMJ* 1977; **ii:** 44.
7 Jolly R. Medical hazards of air travel. *BMJ* 1977; **ii:** 637–8.
8 Lawrie J. Medical responsibilities of airlines. *BMJ* 1981; **292:** 320.
9 Hays MB. Physicians and airline medical emergencies. *Aviat Space Environ Med* 1977; **48:** 468–70.
10 Federal Aviation Administration. Emergency medical equipment requirement. *Fed Reg* 1986; **51:** 1218–23.
11 Hordinsky JR, George MH. Response capability during civil air carrier inflight medical emergencies. *Aviat Space Environ Med* 1989; **60:** 1211–14.
12 MacLaren RB. In-flight medical care by flight attendants—an assessment of overall needs. *Preprints of the 1982 meeting of the Aerospace Medical Association.* Washington, DC: Aerospace Medical Association, 1982: 305–6.
13 Davies GRW, Degotardi PR. Inflight medical facilities. *Aviat Space Environ Med* 1982; **53:** 694–700.
14 Lavernhe J, Lafontaine E, Lequesne M. Transportation of patients in commercial aircraft. *Aerospace Med* 1967; **38:** 525–7.
15 Anonymous. Illness in the clouds (Editorial). *BMJ* 1975; **i:** 295.
16 Schocken V, Lederer LG. Unscheduled landings for medical reasons: a five year survey of the experience at American Airlines. In: Busby DE, ed. *Recent advances in aerospace medicine.* Dordrecht, Holland: Reidel Publishing Co, 1970: 126–9.
17 Cummins RO, Schubach JA. Frequency and types of medical emergencies among commercial air travellers. *JAMA* 1989; **261:** 1295–9.
18 Speizer C, Rennie CJ et al. Prevalence of in-flight medical emergencies on commercial airlines. *Ann Emerg Med* 1989; **18:** 53–6.
19 Cummins RO, Chapman PJC, Chamberlain DA, Schubach JA. In-flight deaths during commercial air travel: how big is the problem? *JAMA* 1988; **259:** 1983–8.
20 Stoner DL, Cooke JP. Intratracheal cuffs and aeromedical evacuation. *Anesthesiology* 1974; **41:** 302–6.
21 American Medical Association commission on emergency medical services. Medical aspects of transportation aboard commercial aircarft. *JAMA* 1982; **247:** 1007–11.
22 Moylan JA, Pruitt BA. Aeromedical transportation. *JAMA* 1973; **224:** 1271–3.
23 Mohler SR, Nicogossian A, Margulies RA. Emergency medicine and the airline passenger. *Aviat Space Environ Med* 1980; **51:** 918–22.
24 Aerospace Medical Association. Resolution 2: Minutes of the 1982 business meeting. *Aviat Space Environ Med* 1982; **53:** 861–4.
25 Thompson LJ. Who should treat medical emergencies on commercial airlines. *Aviat Med Q* 1987; **1:** 125–9.

26 Millett DP. Final report of the sub-committee on the training of flight attendants in first aid. *Aviat Space Environ Med* 1988; **59:** 992–3.

2
Legal aspects of inflight emergencies

It is not what a lawyer tells me I may do; but what humanity, reason, and justice, tell me I ought to do.

Edmund Burke (1729–1797)

Medical emergencies occurring in passenger aircraft and the part that a doctor who might be on board could be called on to play were discussed in chapter 1. When first published, the discussion awoke an interest, in some cases a nagging fear, in the minds of some practitioners with regard to the medicolegal implications of such a predicament.

An authoritative guide is clearly required to spell out the exact implications of every dilemma that could develop. Alas, this is impossible not only in the context of air travel, but also in any parallel problem that might occur on the ground. Were it not so there would be no need for lawyers and judges. All that can be sensibly afforded are some general principles that are likely to be relevant to such circumstances.

British registered aircraft

Because the number of variables in international travel is almost infinite it is best to consider the most straightforward problem and assume that in a British owned and registered aircraft, flying within the United Kingdom, a British subject resident within the country becomes ill and is treated by a doctor who is a fellow passenger. What then are the liabilities, given that the person responding is fully registered to practise medicine in the UK? The solution is also straightforward, and the responsibility and obligations no different from those occurring daily in a doctor's life. The physician will be expected to act with the same reasonable professional skill as on the ground but within the physical restraints—such as limited space, noise, and basic equipment—that inflight conditions impose. The doctor's judgement must always ultimately rest on the patient's best interest, which may not always accord with the convenience of other passengers. He or she would have to remember to act only within the ambit of their own professional skills and not—if an alternative exists—exceed them.

A doctor coming forward as a result of a call for help from the crew, rather than volunteering services direct to a fellow passenger, will technically be acting on behalf of the aircraft operators. This raises another facet of this apparently simple problem and concerns the responsibility of the airlines themselves. They cannot be held responsible for the doctor's professional actions but they must, through the cabin staff, take reasonable care to ensure that so far as it lies within their power this volunteer is a bona fide medical practitioner and not, as has occurred, an impostor. There is a clear duty of care on them to do what they can to check this point, and it is equally clear that such inquiries may well give offence to the doctor concerned. Even if documents, such as a passport, are available and even if these can be requested and produced without the appearance of overzealous suspicion they may be inconclusive. Many who are not medical practitioners use the style of "doctor".

One of the peculiarities of inflight illness is that a basic question to be answered must always be whether the flight can be continued to its destination or whether a premature diversionary landing has to be made. The latter decision may not be popular with anyone, but needs to be made as early as possible, in relation to the fact that the patient's apparent condition may well be one with which a doctor may be entirely unfamiliar after perhaps a lifetime's work in a narrow specialty. Only the doctor will know his or her limitations and experience and will, in order to avoid blame, have to act and advise strictly within the limits of their competence, and must not exceed this if another and safer course is open. On other occasions, when no diversion is possible—such as in long overwater sectors— doctors have no such escape and must do their best. In such circumstances the physician must, therefore, make two decisions, each with its own responsibility: first, that he or she is competent to deal with the circumstances and second to act with reasonable care within that competence.

American registered aircraft

Even the apparently simple problem is not without its nuances, but most will not be as clear cut as this. For example, the passenger, although resident in the United Kingdom, may in fact be an American national or the doctor may be travelling in an aircraft that is registered in another country. The variables are almost infinite and the straightforward principles of English or Scottish law may not apply, as other codes of law may be effective, and the natural inclination of an English court to be sympathetic to a doctor coming forward to help at a time of crisis may not be present. In some other countries, and in particular the United States, the public in general (and therefore the patient population also) is much more litigious, especially where personal injury cases are concerned: in some countries the "ambulance chasing" lawyer is a reality. If the emergency concerns an American passenger, or takes place on an American registered aircraft, an action could be brought in an American court. Two points need explanation.

First, under United States law it is perfectly ethical and normal for a lawyer to act on a contingency basis—that is, taking up any case in which damages may be awarded and agree a fee on a percentage of such damages: no damages, no fee. Many people ascribe the large amount of litigation in some American states to this contingency fee system.

Second, in the United Kingdom the level of damages is always determined by a judge, but this is not the case in the United States, where a civil jury determines the award and the sums involved are often vastly in excess of any yet awarded in the United Kingdom. Because of this, many doctors in the United States and elsewhere would think twice before volunteering their services in an emergency, and might even consider it prudent not to intervene at all. This is a point of view which is understandable if uncommendable.

Good samaritan legislation

As a direct consequence of this problem attempts have been made to introduce a "good samaritan act" in the United States. Such a bill was introduced to congress some time ago by representative Carl Pursell, and sought to relieve any doctor, registered nurse, or aircraft employee who rendered medical attention to an ill or injured person on board an aircraft of any civil liabilities, except in the case of gross or wilful negligence. The bill did not become law because, no matter how laudable its intentions may have been, its object was to reduce the amount of legislation, and its effect would thus have been to reduce the work of lawyers in a country in which an exceptionally strong legal lobby exists. During 1983, senator Goldwater introduced an inflight emergencies bill to congress which included two main provisions. The first required a certain standard of medical equipment to be carried on board passenger aircraft with 30 seats or more, and the second provided a good samaritan clause similar to that in the Pursell proposals. This predictably met considerable opposition from the legal lobby and seemed stalled until, quite suddenly, it was approved and enacted on 1 August 1985. This agreement, however, was secured only after considerable negotiation (in effect, "plea bargaining") during which specific exclusion clauses were inserted, thereby neatly emasculating the bill in its scope and usefulness. The bill provided that those who, in good faith, rendered emergency medical care on board an aircraft should not be liable for any civil damages as a result of any act or omission, but it then went on to lay down that this defence was available neither to the air carriers themselves nor to doctors: hence the effective emasculation. Indeed, the chief negotiator for the legal lobby explained that such people would be carrying adequate liability insurance of their own: they would therefore, it is to be supposed, be legitimate targets!

In the absence at present of good samaritan legislation anywhere in the world the doctor is, therefore, in a position of being bound by that code of law which applies according to circumstances, and the inherent changes of liability will therefore vary greatly and depend on many factors. This being so, a doctor can act only with the best possible skill and care that he or she can muster, and may ultimately have to rely on help from a professional defence society. It has to be understood, however, that there is no contractual obligation between such an organisation and its members automatically to undertake each case presented. The three defence societies in the United Kingdom have acquired an enviable reputation of standing by their members whenever there is a case that impugns a doctor's professional conduct, but they specifically exclude from their cover any litigation in the United States resulting from a member's activities, wherever these may have taken place. This being so, and despite the fact that no case has so far arisen in which a British doctor has been sued under United

States jurisdiction for an act taking place in an aircraft, the need for effective good samaritan legislation is clearly pressing.

Training of cabin staff

If reasonable skill and competence are shown then, regardless of where the act takes place, there should be no case to answer, but this does not mean that there is nothing to fear. Such hazards as possible vexatious litigation—conditions as they obtain in the United States (and the exclusion that the defence societies exercise in respect of that country) and the uncertainty about jurisdiction that may well exist in international travel—must mean that doctors may be backward in coming forward when assistance is sought other than on board a British registered aircraft. Even here the matter may be complicated because certain circumstances—for example, a patient who is an American citizen—may bring with them the right for a claim to be made other than in British courts. Because of all these difficulties, it is little wonder that opinion in most airline medical departments is that the best service to the sick or injured passenger can probably be achieved by greatly improved training of a small number of cabin staff, up to something approaching paramedic standards. Such training would enable them to deal competently with a much greater range of inflight emergencies, which is one of the recommendations for improvement suggested in chapter 1. Given the type of illness or accident that tends to occur during flight, the variable quality of the response that a call for assistance may evoke, and the reservations that some doctors feel in undertaking something that they believe might have unusual repercussions, many are convinced that this is the logical step for airlines, and international carriers in particular, to take; as indeed many are now doing. Nevertheless, until this is fully achieved, and even after, the doctor faced with this dilemma must first decide what is the best course of action to take, based on his or her skill and judgement, and then to act in the best manner possible in the light of all the circumstances prevailing. No one can do more.

3
Fitness to travel by air

I always love to begin a journey on Sundays, because I shall have the prayers of the church, to preserve all that travel by land, or by water

Jonathan Swift (1667–1745)

Commercial aviation has added a new dimension to everyday travel and for most passengers it is a safe and efficient method of transport, although not entirely without potential medical problems (of a less serious nature than those discussed in chapter 1), even for those who begin their journey fully fit. For some patients, however, flying means exposure to additional medical risks that may not be apparent to them or to their doctors. This chapter discusses various aspects which determine whether patients are fit to fly as fare paying passengers on civil airlines, and some other matters of importance to all.

General considerations

The prime concerns of an airline are the safe transportation of the public and the maintenance of a high standard of service. These objectives may be affected adversely by the carriage of sick passengers. For example, an unescorted pyschotic patient could be a grave threat to the safety of an aircraft and its passengers, or a patient whose disease is well controlled on the ground may become acutely ill when subjected to the physiological conditions of flight. Cabin staff are trained in basic first aid, but in some cases expert medical attention may be obtained only if the aircaft makes an unscheduled landing. Apart from being extremely expensive for the airline, such a diversion will also cause delay and inconvenience to other passengers. For these reasons, airlines (not unreasonably) reserve the right to refuse passage to those who are not medically fit to travel by air. Most major carriers, therefore, have a medical department to advise on a patient's suitability for air travel and, if feasible, to make special arrangements, such as giving extra help for passengers in wheelchairs and accommodating stretcher cases. Provision of these extra services requires prior notification of the patient's condition to the airline, and may incur additional charges. British Airways and most other airlines welcome inquiries from doctors, and encourage the use of a simple form, the MEDIF, developed by the International Air Transport Association. The form is available from travel agents or direct from the airlines, and should be completed by both patient (Part 1) and doctor (Part 2) so that all relevant information can be obtained in advance. Probably because of ignorance of this system, too many medically compromised passengers arrive for travel unannounced.[1]

Circumstances sometimes dictate that travel has to be undertaken at short notice, and many airlines also have a specialist medical officer available at all times to answer urgent inquiries from doctors with problem cases. For British Airways such inquiries should be directed to the medical officer, British Airways Health Services, Queen's Building, Heathrow Airport, Hounslow, Middlesex TW6 2JA (telephone 081 562 7070). The advice given by the airline will be determined by physiological and specific medical considerations.

Physiological considerations

A patient with a disease which will be affected adversely by the hypoxia, pressure changes produced by altitude, or both will commonly be advised not to fly (see also chapter 5).

Conditions adversely affected by hypoxia

Respiratory diseases—At a cabin altitude of 1829 m (6000 ft) the alveolar partial pressure of oxygen falls from 13·7 kPa (103 mmHg) to 10·3 kPa (77 mmHg), but the sigmoid shape of the haemoglobin oxygen dissociation curve reflects the fact that the oxygen saturation of haemoglobin will have been reduced by only 3% at that altitude. Some older aircraft are still flying with a maximum cabin altitude of 2438 m (8000 ft), but even at this height saturation will have fallen to only about 90%. Such reductions present no problems to the healthy passenger but may exacerbate certain medical conditions, the most obvious of which are those where pulmonary function is impaired. Thus, in patients with chronic bronchitis, emphysema, bronchiectasis, and cor pulmonale where oxygenation is already compromised, exposure to altitude may result in severe tissue hypoxia.[2] Most of these patients may be transported safely provided that supplementary oxygen is available during the flight; and a ground level partial pressure of oxygen (Po_2) of $\leqslant 6.25$ kPa (50 mmHg) is a good indication that supplementary oxygen should be used.[3] The use of 100% oxygen may, however, worsen some cases because it may remove the hypoxic drive to ventilation essential to many patients, with consequent hypoventilation and carbon dioxide retention. The measurement of blood gases in flight may be desirable, but it is impractical on board an aircraft. With ear oximetry, however, haemoglobin saturation may be monitored relatively easily even in flight.[4] In general, dyspnoea at rest is a contraindication to flight, and patients with poor exercise tolerance (dyspnoea after walking 50 m on level ground) require further assessment[2] with full pulmonary function tests and a trial of 100% oxygen. Recent evidence suggests that although a low preflight arterial Po_2 level provides a useful pointer to likely inflight problems, the additional use of pulmonary function tests, and particularly the FEV_1, is even more valuable; and it may even be possible to improve performance by intensive preflight therapy.[5] Several other simple measures will improve the lot of those with chronic obstructive airway disease (and indeed any other passenger with a preflight medical problem), including early unflustered arrival and check-in, prompt notification to airline staff of potential problems, use of wheelchairs to prevent undue exertion, and avoidance of seats anywhere near a smoking area.

Well controlled asthma should not be a contraindication to flight,[6] but once again careful planning is essential: additional inhalers and other medications should be carried, and precipitating stressors avoided as far as possible. Similarly, patients with mild cystic fibrosis, as evidenced by adequate pulmonary function, should not encounter problems; while those whose respiratory function is compromised should follow the guidelines for supplementary oxygen outlined above. Patients who produce large amounts of offensive sputum may not be permitted to fly, however, despite satisfactory ventilation, because of disturbance to other passengers:[7] a commercial consideration that applies to some other medical conditions—for example, urinary or faecal incontinence, or gross disfigurement.

Anaemias—Severe anaemia, usually defined as a haemoglobin concentration of less than 7·5 g dl^{-1}, is a relative contraindication to air travel[2] depending on the chronicity of the condition and the length of the flight to be undertaken. Transfusion before flight may be required, and the airline medical department should be consulted so that supplementary oxygen is readily available on board the aircraft. Cases of sickling crisis precipitated by flight have been reported[8] and, although hypoxia is usually the major predisposing factor, prolonged sitting causes abdominal compression and venestasis, which are also conducive to the development of sickling. The particular groups at risk are those with sickle cell haemoglobin C disease and sickle cell β thalassaemia.[9] Affected subjects should be advised to avoid air travel, but if this is not possible additional oxygen should be readily available. Sickle cell trait—that is, the heterozygous carrier state—is no longer a serious risk because of cabin pressurisation. Surprisingly, patients with sickle cell anaemia are at little risk in pressurised aircraft, possibly because of autosplenectomy.[8]

Cardiovascular diseases—Patients who have poor cardiac reserve require careful assessment before flight because they may be unable to tolerate the slight reduction in inspired oxygen tension which occurs at high cabin altitudes.[10] As a guideline, those who are able to walk about 80 m and to climb 10–12 stairs without symptoms should be able to fly without incident,[11] but uncontrolled cardiac failure is a contraindication to flight. However, in a study of 25 patients admitted to hospital after collapsing at Heathrow airport with conditions affecting the cardiovascular system, myocardial insufficiency tended to occur on the ground rather than in the air.[12] The stress and exhaustion imposed by air travel seem to be at least as important as other predisposing factors such as hypoxia during flight. In another study of 615 passengers with established cardiovascular and respiratory disease, those with myocardial ischaemia did not have a significantly greater number of problems than in the survey population as a whole.[13] The incidence of complications was, however, much higher than in a poorly defined control group. Interestingly, the number of episodes of angina in flight was more than double that on the ground but, in this study, help with documentation and baggage at embarkation and disembarkation kept "ground stress" to a minimum. Of patients with a history of myocardial infarction, those who had suffered a recent infarct (less than 2 months before flight) or a history of multiple infarcts had a significantly higher incidence of problems during flight than those with an intermediate history—that is, an infarct 2–6 months before flying. Thus, recent myocardial infarction should be regarded as a contraindication to air travel. But, as many patients wish to convalesce abroad, British Airways recommends as a compromise that patients in uncomplicated cases do not fly for a minimum of 2 weeks after an infarct.

Neurological diseases—Hypoxia may affect patients who have had a recent cerebral infarction, but problems are less likely to arise as the interval after the stroke increases:[13] a minimum of 3 weeks after the acute episode is the recommended interval before flight. Atherosclerosis may have already diminished cerebral oxygenation in the elderly passenger and, although this may not be severe enough to produce symptoms on the ground, the mild hypoxia at cabin altitude may tip the balance towards frank cerebral hypoxia. As such patients often become confused, they should be escorted by a friend or relative. As a general rule, patients who tend to become confused at night are likely to develop similar symptoms during flight. Age alone is not, however, a contraindication to flying as a passenger.[6] Epileptics may be more liable to seizures while travelling by air because of several predisposing factors including hypoxia, hyperventilation, fatigue, and stress. Poorly controlled epileptics should be advised to increase their medication 24 hours before flight and maintain a high dose until arrival at their ultimate destination when the dosage may be reduced gradually. During long flights the patient's usual routine may be disturbed by time changes and medication should be continued on a regular basis, usually by the patient remaining on home time throughout the journey and adjusting the drug regimen on arrival.

Other factors—The effects of hypoxia may be worsened by several other factors, especially by cigarettes and alcohol. Patients who are at risk from hypoxia should therefore be advised to abstain from both habits before and during flight. Even so, hypoxia may still be an overwhelming physiological challenge at certain destinations; a patient with chronic bronchitis is ill advised to convalesce in Mexico City, for example, which lies 2273 m (7460 ft) above sea level!

Conditions adversely affected by pressure changes

Gas taken to 1829 m (6000 ft) above sea level will, if free to do so, increase its volume by about 30% because of reduced atmospheric pressure. Air contained within body cavities also undergoes this physical change—hence the need to 'clear' one's ears during descent (see also chapter 5). Severe otic and sinus barotrauma are fairly uncommon medical complications of flying, but otitis media and sinusitis greatly increase the risk of such damage: those who are affected should be advised not to fly during the acute stage of the illness.[14] If travel is unavoidable, a nasal decongestant is a useful addition to hand luggage, and many people include such medication as a routine when flying.

Patients who have had recent middle ear surgery are particularly at risk and should not fly until the middle ear cavity is dry and normally aerated.[2] Patients who have undergone stapedectomy also require special attention because the prosthesis may be driven into the labyrinth by pressure changes, thus causing vertigo and cochlear failure.[15] Specialist advice must be obtained for these patients before flight is allowed; and even then they must be warned to 'clear' their ears early and frequently during descent.[16]

Expansion of gas within the gastrointestinal tract will manifest on ascent in healthy passengers by a tightening of clothing at the waist, especially if gas-producing food and drinks such as beans, brassica vegetables, curries, and alcohol or carbonated beverages are consumed. Moderation in gastronomic and drinking habits is therefore recommended, along with loosely fitting and comfortable clothes, although such expansion is usually innocuous.

Gas expansion may, however, cause problems after abdominal surgery because of dehiscence of the abdominal wound or, more particularly, disruption of a bowel anastomosis. At least 10 days should elapse between abdominal surgery, however minor, and flight, but this time limit should be extended if the postoperative recovery was complicated by paralytic ileus. Recent gastrointestinal haemorrhage may be reactivated by distension of the bowel so that flying should not be undertaken for at least 3 weeks; motion sickness could further aggravate the problem. Those with ileostomies or colostomies may need to vent the increased volume of gastrointestinal gas and should be warned to take extra bags and dressings in their hand luggage.[2]

Air may be introduced into the thoracic cavity during thoracic surgery, and its expansion may result in respiratory embarrassment, so 3 weeks is also the recommended interval between major chest surgery and air travel. For the same reason patients with

35

pneumothorax should not fly until it has been confirmed radiologically that the lung has re-expanded fully.[7]

Air trapped within the cranium during air encephalography is an absolute contraindication to air travel,[2] and at least 7 days should be allowed for the air to be absorbed. Similar restrictions apply to patients who have a skull fracture extending into a sinus or the middle ear cavity through which air may have entered the cranium.[17] Trapped air may also produce problems after eye injury and surgery.[7]

When air trapped within plaster casts expands the enclosed limb may be sufficiently compressed to cause ischaemia.[18] Casts should therefore be split before a flight if the underlying soft tissues are still oedematous, especially if the flight is going to be lengthy. Passengers with plasters extending above the knee may also create problems by obstructing aisles or emergency exits. Often the only solution is for the passenger to travel first class, where more leg room is available, or to travel on a stretcher.

Psychiatric disorders and fear of flying

Flying often provokes anxiety and presents a person with many unusual stimuli including noise, vibration, disruption of sleep, the proximity of strangers, and a change of location. Unexpected delays, often during transit stops in foreign countries, may cause further disturbances both mental and physical. For these reasons patients with psychiatric disorders, who may have been living a regular and undisturbed routine for many years in a sheltered environment, need careful consideration before being allowed to fly. And, because of the need to ensure the comfort and safety of other passengers, airlines usually expect a psychiatric patient to be escorted by a relative or a qualified mental nurse, the level of expertise depending on the severity of the illness. At worst the patient may require constant sedation, but the agent should be carefully chosen. For example, drugs with anticholinergic activity may predispose to increased intestinal gas, which—when aggravated by altitude—may reduce the mobility of the diaphragm and impair respiration.[19] Sedated patients are also more likely to develop barotrauma and, because of the risk of deep vein thrombosis and nerve palsy due to prolonged sitting, they should be restrained in a supine position on long journeys. For this purpose an aircraft stretcher can be provided after consultation with the airline's medical department. Several hundreds of stretcher cases are carried by British Airways each year (1160 worldwide in 1992/93), usually for reasons other than chemical sedation, but the extra room needed to accommodate a stretcher (each requires the allocation of nine seats) has to be paid for by the passenger.[20]

Up to 15% of the population is estimated to have a true fear of flying which prevents affected individuals from ever setting foot in an airport, let alone on an aircraft. Such a flying phobia causes much misery and can present great professional and social difficulties. Treatment programmes based on cognitive-behavioural techniques are now available, and are usually conducted by clinical psychologists either with or without the direct involvement of an airline. The courses, which are often effective in the short term, usually consist of a ground-based phase of behavioural therapy followed by a "desensitising" flight in the company of the professional counsellor.

Other preflight conditions

Diabetes mellitus

Diabetic patients often ask their doctors for advice on air travel, particularly when undertaking long journeys through several time zones. Generally, such passengers should remain on home time throughout their journey for both meals and medication, and adjust to local time only after arrival at their destination. With careful planning, however, fine tuning the insulin regimen is possible; and a recent study suggested that an increase during westward flights of 2–4% of the daily insulin dose per hour of time zone shift and a similar decrease during eastward flights maintained good glycaemic control.[21] The additional requirement during westward travel was achieved by normal doses supplemented by injections of short acting insulin with meals; while slightly reduced normal doses were used during eastward travel. Diabetics who are prone to airsickness should be given appropriate prophylactic medication such as hyoscine (0·6 mg).

As with any other patient taking regular medication, diabetics should be reminded to carry it in their hand luggage rather than to be embarrassed in flight by realising that it is secured in the cargo hold. It is also advisable to carry a covering letter from their doctor giving details of treatment and a means of seeking further information.

Pregnancy

Although flying is unlikely to be harmful to a normal pregnancy, an aircraft is not an ideal delivery suite. Most airlines will therefore not carry passengers after 35 weeks of pregnancy or, in the case of domestic flights, after 36 weeks. Of course, premature labour is always a possibility, or the pregnancy may be undeclared: four live deliveries occurred on British Airways flights in 1991/92. Some countries refuse entry to passengers in advanced stages of pregnancy, so pregnant women should check the immigration rules of the country to be visited. They should also be aware that they are at increased risk of the problems of orthostasis (see below) and that anaemia of pregnancy may give rise to hypoxia at altitude (see above).[22]

Neonates

Babies should not fly during the first 48 hours of life because some alveoli will not have expanded and a degree of ventilation-perfusion inequality will result. Even a healthy neonate may have an arterial oxygen partial pressure of 8·7–10·7 kPa (65–80 mmHg) that would be worsened by increasing altitude.[18]

Human immunodeficiency virus

The emergence on a global scale of the acquired immune deficiency syndrome (AIDS) epidemic has inevitably raised several issues relating to human immunodeficiency virus (HIV) infection and international travel. The World Health Organization, in reporting the findings of its consultation on the subject, identified three particular problems.[23] The first was the possibility of screening all international travellers, which, it was realistically concluded, would be cripplingly expensive and unlikely to achieve any lasting effect in retarding the spread of the disease. The second was the public conveyance of those infected with HIV. The consultation stated categorically that the "use of any public conveyance (for example, train, bus, airplane, boat) by persons infected with the human immunodeficiency virus *does not* create a risk of infection for others sharing the same conveyance." This statement was applied equally to "healthy carriers" and to those with clinical manifestations of HIV infection, including AIDS. It was concluded, therefore, that "there is no specific reason to limit the use of public conveyances by HIV-infected persons." The third aspect considered by the consultation was the dissemination of information. It was recommended that educational material should be made widely available (through travel agencies, accommodation booking agencies, and airlines as well as through the more traditional medical sources) to increase awareness of how HIV is transmitted and how the risks of transmission can be minimised.[23] The difficult problem of aircrew and cabin staff infected with HIV is discussed in chapter 10.

Other inflight conditions

Motion sickness

Airsickness is rarely a problem because commercial aircraft fly at altitudes above the worst turbulence. But should it occur prevention by pharmacological means is a realistic approach for most passengers (see chapter 7). For one very small group of patients, however, the development of motion sickness could be fatal: those with permanent wiring of the jaws following faciomaxillary surgery should not be allowed to travel unless the fixation has a quick release mechanism. The patient should be familiar with the mechanism and realise the dangers of aspirating vomit.

Orthostasis

The sedentary nature of air travel predisposes to postural oedema and, as a consequence, to the possibility of deep vein thrombosis and pulmonary embolism. Both conditions are more likely in those with a history of cardiovascular disease (such as pre-existing venestasis, heart failure or trauma) and during pregnancy, but even the young and those with no predisposing factors can be affected. Furthermore, although more likely to develop during very long journeys, these conditions can develop during relatively short flights (3–4 hours) and their presentation delayed for days afterwards. Cramped seating, lack of mobility, and dehydration compounded by excessive alcohol consumption have all been cited as contributory causes and have given rise to the term "economy class syndrome".[24] All passengers should therefore be advised to take regular walks about the cabin, and to perform leg exercises when seated. If possible, the legs should be elevated. Both smoking and alcohol exacerbate hypoxia and increase blood viscosity, and should be avoided. Those known to be at risk should be considered for low dose aspirin therapy.[24]

Jet lag (see also transmeridian travel, chapter 9)

The endogenous circadian system, in which over 50 physiological and psychological rhythms have now been identified, is known to be affected by many environmental factors including clock hour, light and dark, and temperature although many of the rhythms continue in the absence of such cues, albeit usually with slightly prolonged periodicity.[25] The environmental factors facilitate entrainment or phasing of the rhythms, and are known as synchronisers or *zeitgebers* (time givers). Travel across time zones outstrips the ability of synchronisers to entrain rhythms and desynchronisation occurs: this is responsible for the syndrome known as jet lag, because circadian rhythms need a finite period to become re-entrained to local time (usually estimated at about 1 day per time zone crossed).[26] Westward travel is generally considered to be better tolerated than eastward,[27] possibly because the endogenous system—with a natural periodicity in most subjects of about 25 hours—is more able to adapt to the longer "day" encountered during westward flight.[28] Many methods of reducing or preventing the consequences of jet lag have been proposed (suggesting that none is entirely effective), including careful preflight manipulation of sleep and eating patterns, but these are impracticable for most people. Although a "jet lag pill" is theoretically possible, greater knowledge of the neurotransmitter mechanisms involved in entrainment will be needed before such sophisticated pharmacological manipulation is a reality.[29]

Various simple methods can, however, be employed by passengers to minimise the effects, such as sleeping on the aircraft (with or without the benefit of a short acting hypnotic), avoiding heavy meals and excessive alcohol, avoiding important commitments for at least 24 hours after arrival, and generally being aware of an inevitable reduction in physical and mental performance for a few days. Temazepam (20 mg) has recently been shown to have a beneficial effect on sleep and alertness after transmeridian travel, although it had no effect on performance and did not alter the rate of re-entrainment of physiological rhythms.[30] The aetiology of the effects of jet lag—sleep disturbances, disruption of other body functions such as feeding and bowel habit, general discomfort, and reduced psychomotor efficiency—has been the subject of much investigation which has largely concentrated on underlying hormonal variations.[28,31]

Terminal illnesses

Terminally ill patients often wish to travel by air, to spend their last days at a specific location or to visit relatives living abroad. Airlines consider such requests with compassion but have to refuse patients who may die during flight. Of over 700 passengers examined by the medical department of Air France over 2 years, 17 were not permitted to embark; nine of these had an illness which was likely to result in death during flight.[32] Such an incident may cause great difficulties for the bereaved family, who have not only to arrange for the return of the body from a foreign country but also have to deal with subtle legal questions. For example, which country has to be satisfied as to the cause of death when an American citizen dies while overflying French airspace in a British aircraft that later lands in Bahrain?

Aeromedical evacuation

So far the contraindications to patients flying by civil airlines have largely been determined by commercial considerations as much as by medical ones. For example, patients with air in the cranium may not fly in commercial aircraft because the cabin altitude is unlikely to be lower than 1829 m (6000 ft) and decompression to higher altitude is always a risk. If geography permits, such a patient may be carried on an aircraft flying at a guaranteed maximum ambient altitude of 1219 m (4000 ft), an uneconomic altitude for airline operations. If treatment is urgent, however, agencies experienced in aeromedical transport will have to be used—see chapter 4.

1 McIntosh IB. The disabled and handicapped traveller. *Travel Med International* 1992; **10**: 101–4.
2 Green RL. The carriage of invalid passengers by air. *Br J Hosp Med* 1977; **17**: 32–7.
3 Miles JF, Ayres JG. Travel and respiratory disease. *Travel Med International* 1990; **8**: 147–50.
4 Cissik JH, Yochey CC, Byrd RB. Evaluation of the Hewlett-Packard ear oximeter for use during routine air transport of patients. *Aviat Space Environ Med* 1981; **52**: 312–14.
5 Dillard TA, Berg BW, Rajagopal KR, Dooley JW, Mehr WJ. Hypoxaemia during air travel in patients with chronic obstructive airway disease. *Ann Intern Med* 1989; **111**: 362–7.

6 Committee on medical criteria of the Aerospace Medical Association. Medical criteria for passenger flying. *J Aviat Med* 1961; **32:** 369–82.
7 Bergin K. Transport of invalids by air. *BMJ* 1967; **iii:** 539–43.
8 Green RL, Huntsman RG, Serjeant GR. The sickle-cell and altitude. *BMJ* 1971; **iv:** 593–5.
9 Green RL, Huntsman RG, Serjeant GR. Sickle-cell and altitude. *BMJ* 1972; **i:** 803–4.
10 Jackson F. The heart at high altitude. *Br Heart J* 1968; **30:** 291–4.
11 Peters ASR. Carriage of invalids by air. *J R Coll Physicians Lond* 1978; **12:** 136–42.
12 Beighton PH, Richards PR. Cardiovascular disease in air travellers. *Br Heart J* 1968; **30:** 367–72.
13 Richards PR. The effects of air travel on passengers with cardiovascular and respiratory disease. *Practitioner* 1973; **210:** 232–41.
14 King PF. Fit to fly? Some common problems in otolaryngology. *Aviat Med Q* 1988; **2:** 19–29.
15 King PF. Otorhinolaryngology. In: Ernsting J, King PF, eds. *Aviation medicine*, 2nd edn. London: Butterworths, 1988: 656.
16 Moser M. Fitness of civil aviation passengers to fly after ear surgery. *Aviat Space Environ Med* 1990; **61:** 735–7.
17 Ellingson HV. Aerial transportation of patients. In: Randel HW, ed. *Aerospace medicine*, 2nd edn. Baltimore: Williams and Wilkins Company, 1971: 602–13.
18 Parsons CJ, Bobechko WP. Aeromedical transport: its hidden problems. *Can Med Assoc J* 1982; **126:** 237–43.
19 Jones DR. Aeromedical transportation of psychiatric patients: historical review and present management. *Aviat Space Environ Med* 1980; **51:** 709–16.
20 Green RL, Mooney SE. Carriage of invalid passengers by civil airlines. In: Ernsting J, King PF, eds. *Aviation medicine*, 2nd edn. London: Butterworths, 1988: 553.
21 Sane T, Koivisto VA, Nikkanen P, Pelkonen R. Adjustment of insulin dosage during long-distance flights. *BMJ* 1990; **301:** 421–2.
22 Barry M, Bia F. Pregnancy and travel. *JAMA* 1989; **261:** 728–31.
23 WHO Special Programme on AIDS. *Report on the consultation on international travel and HIV infection.* Geneva: World Health Organization, 1987 (WHO/SPA/GLO/87.1).
24 Cruickshank JM, Gorlin R, Jennett B. Air travel and thrombotic episodes: the economy class syndrome. *Lancet* 1988; **ii:** 497–8.
25 Mills JN, Minors DS, Waterhouse MJ. The circadian rhythms of human subjects without timepieces or indications of the alteration of day and night. *J Physiol (Lond)* 1974; **240:** 567–94.
26 McFarland RA. Influence of changing time zones on air crews and passengers. *Aerospace Med* 1974; **45:** 648–58.
27 Elliot AN, Mills JN, Minors DS, Waterhouse JM. Effect of simulated time zone shifts upon plasma corticosteroid rhythms. *J Physiol (Lond)* 1971; **217:** 50P.
28 Arendt J, Marks V. Physiological changes underlying jet lag. *BMJ* 1982; **284:** 144–6.
29 Redfern PH. Can pharmacological agents be used effectively in alleviation of jet-lag? *Drugs* 1992; **43:** 146–53.
30 Donaldson E, Kennaway DJ. Effects of temazepam on sleep, performance, and rhythmic 6-sulphatoxymelatonin and cortisol after transmeridian travel. *Aviat Space Environ Med* 1991; **62:** 654–60.
31 Désir D, Van Cauter E, Fang VS *et al.* Effects of "jet lag" on hormonal patterns. 1. Procedures, variations in total plasma proteins, and disruption of adrenocorticotropin cortisol periodicity. *J Clin Endocrinol Metab* 1981; **52:** 628–41.
32 Lavernhe J, Lafontaine E, Lequesne M. Transportation of patients in commercial aircraft. *Aerospace Med* 1967; **38:** 525–7.

4
Transport of patients by air

The physician must look beyond the picture, now widely cherished, of the lonely, great-hearted doctor, bowed impotent beside the dying child. Modern transportation, modern methods of diagnosis and treatment, have made that picture as obsolete as the village blacksmith at his charcoal forge.

William Dock (b. 1898)

The history of aeromedical transportation is almost as long as the history of powered flight itself. The earliest recorded evacuation of wounded casualties by aircraft took place during the first world war (1915), when twelve Serbian patients were carried in French aircraft.[1] As aviation technology progressed, so did the awareness of the potential for the use of aircraft as airborne ambulances. Although in the 1920s military aircraft were used for disaster relief missions in the United States and during the same period the Royal Air Force operated an air ambulance service within a 100 mile radius of Halton in the United Kingdom, it was not until 1933 that the first British civilian air ambulance service was instigated. Serving the Scottish isles, the descendant of this service still operates today, carrying the sick and injured from the remote islands of Scotland to the mainland. Long distance high altitude aeromedical evacuation, however, was pioneered by the Luftwaffe during the Spanish civil war (1936–41). Using trimotor Junkers JU 52 aircraft, missions lasting up to 10 hours were flown at an altitude of 5486 m (18 000 ft). The second world war, by necessity, heralded rapid advancement and created much work for the newly formed military casualty evacuation (casevac) organisations. In the latter years of the conflict more than 90% of allied casualties were evacuated by air from all theatres.

The military continued to dominate advances in aeromedical transportation in the immediate postwar period, particularly in countries which maintained interests and territories overseas. A steady stream of conflicts and minor wars also combined to ensure the continued growth and interest in aeromedical transportation. During the same period, other notable advances made a marked impact.

The first was the development of rotary wing aircraft with their ability to hover and to land and take off from confined spaces. Although first used in the search and rescue role in Burma in 1944, the combat experience of the British in Malaya, the French in Indochina and the United Nations in Korea clearly demonstrated the potential value of helicopters in reducing the mortality rates of battlefield casualties. The Vietnam conflict was, however, to be the definitive proving ground of the helicopter. Dedicated squadrons of turbine-engined Bell UH-1 Iroquois (Huey) casevac helicopters, nicknamed "Dust-Offs", were used for the rapid removal of injured troops from near to the point of wounding (in both the temporal and spatial sense).[2] Development of the Huey was continued during the 10 years of the conflict. It was a fast, manoeuvrable helicopter, with the ability and power to carry four stretchers and a medical team into and out of small clearings with all the constraints imposed by the humidity and heat of the jungle environment. Casualties were then rapidly transported to nearby expert medical care for definitive treatment. This concept was called "scoop and run" and probably accounted, at least partly, for the much lower mortality rate of those wounded in this conflict when compared with those injured in previous wars (table 4.1).[3]

The second phenomenon of major significance was the rapid progress in the technology of mass transportation: bigger and faster passenger carrying aircraft bringing affordable and accessible travel to millions every year. Rapid airline growth in the postwar years and commercial exploitation have brought the furthermost and most exotic corners of the earth within reach of

TABLE 4.1—Battlefield mortality rates*

Conflict	Time (injury–treatment)	Overall mortality rate (%)
World war I	12–18 hours	8·5
World war II	6–12 hours	5·8
Korea	2–4 hours	2·4
Vietnam	65–80 min	1·7

*After Trunkey.[3]

44

the dedicated tourist; not to mention those who travel on business or in the pursuit of adventurous sports.

In the aeromedical role, fixed and rotary wing aircraft can be used in a number of ways (table 4.2), in the combat zone, used as emeregency vehicles, or in the taxi/ferrying role. Many aircraft types are used, each with its advantages and disadvantages according to the requirements of the mission. Outside the military and the emergency medical services (EMS), however, few operators maintain aircraft solely for use in aeromedical transportation, relying rather on the adaptation of existing types as and when the operational requirement arises.

Search and rescue

Fixed wing aircraft have not been used in oversea operations to carry patients since amphibious light aircraft were used during the second world war to retrieve aviators who had ditched or parachuted into the sea. Helicopters, with their ability to lift (winch) survivors directly on board from any environment (and during all but the most severe weather conditions), are now used almost exclusively, whereas long range (high endurance) fixed wing aircraft may be utilised to locate an incident, drop survival equipment, and to act as airborne rescue control and coordination centres.

In the United Kingdom, the entire coastline and the so-called "wilderness areas" (mountains and moorlands) are covered by a network of search and rescue helicopters operated by the Royal Air

TABLE 4.2—Aeromedical transportation missions

Primary	Secondary	Tertiary
Search and rescue	Interhospital transfer	Interhospital transfer
Evacuation from scene of emergency	Battlefield tactical evacuation to next	International repatriation
Transportation of skilled personnel to scene of emergency	echelon of care (within theatre of operations)	Transportation of donor organs
Transportation of equipment and medical matériel to scene of emergency		Battlefield strategic evacuation (out of theatre)
Battlefield scoop and run		

Force, Royal Navy and Coastguard. Most rescues (90%) involve civilian incidents,[4] although the raison d'être for the search and rescue network is the location and retrieval of downed military aircrew and stranded sailors.[5] To cater for this predominantly civilian peacetime role, the service can be activated by the police authorities, and is controlled by two rescue coordination control centres, one in Edinburgh and the other in Plymouth.[6] Similar systems operate in Europe and North America.

Although most commonly used in the scoop and run role, some search and rescue helicopters carry experienced and well equipped medically trained personnel as part of the crew complement. Doctors or flight nurses may also be carried on some missions but, in general, it is advisable that all rescue and retrieval personnel have prior training and experience before undertaking work in the uncomfortable and noisy environment of the helicopter itself, and in the potentially hostile environment of the rescue location.

Military helicopters

Over and above the search and rescue service, other military helicopters may be tasked to aid the civilian community in the event of a disaster or major incident. Such action requires approval and organisation by the relevant defence department and these helicopters, unlike the search and rescue force, are not on permanent standby. The time to activate callout may therefore be long, especially at night and weekends, thereby delaying the start of productive service.

In the battlefield role, it has been shown that helicopters are ideally suited for the rapid collection and removal of patients both in the tactical situation—that is, from the front line (the point of wounding)—and ahead of it (covert operations) and backwards along the evacuation chain through the various echelons of medical care (fig 4.1).[7] Helicopters have also proved invaluable in seaborne operations,[8] for the transfer of casualties between vessels of the Fleet, and from hospital ships to landbased medical facilities or to aeromedical staging facilities for onward transportation.

Civilian helicopters

In Europe, the lessons learned from battlefield casualty evacuation were soon put to good use. Some countries have established

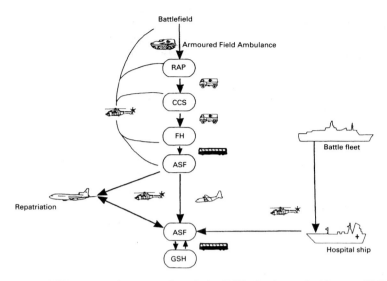

FIG 4.1—Military casualty evacuation chain. RAP, Regimental aid post; CCS, casualty clearing station; FH, field hospital; ASF, aeromedical staging facility; GSH, general surgical hospital.

combined military and civilian networks to cover all major high-ways and special risk areas such as major cities, coastline and mountainous terrain. In the United States, lessons from the Korean and Vietnamese conflicts were quickly learned by the civilian medical authorities. Helicopters were first introduced in Maryland in 1969 to improve patient outcome in what was called the "neglected disease of modern society". This phrase was coined in a report by the US National Research Council which revealed that accidents were the leading cause of death in those under 37 years of age.[9] Since then, there has been a dramatic growth in emergency medical helicopter systems with 160 programmes reported in 1989.[10]

Civilian helicopters may be hospital based or operated by ambulance, fire or police authorities. They may be used for transportation directly to and from the accident scene, or they may be utilized solely for the secondary, but urgent, transfer of high dependency patients,[11] medical supplies or organs for donation. In the former (EMS) role, the responsibility for dispatch and control inevitably lies with the ambulance authority which will have a local protocol driven dispatch system designed to ensure that the EMS helicopter is assigned to the most appropriate missions.[12]

Most EMS helicopters carry a paramedic in addition to the flight crew, although many European (and some North American) EMS helicopters carry a doctor who is trained in advanced prehospital emergency care. In addition, or as an alternative, suitably trained flight nurses are sometimes included as crew members in the United States. The helicopter system may operate in a rural area where the population is sparse, and where there is a low incidence of trauma. In this context, the helicopter is useful to cover large gaps in ambulance cover, especially where there are few hospitals scattered over a wide area.[13] Alternatively, an urban based system is likely to operate in an area of large population yielding a high incidence of trauma where, although appropriate hospitals may be abundant and nearby, traffic congestion impairs rapid evacuation by road.[14]

Of the many controversial issues surrounding the use of helicopters in the EMS role, perhaps none causes so much discussion as the question of prehospital treatment. There are two fundamental concepts, each of which have their vociferous proponents. The first concept is much the same as that used in Vietnam; that is, to reach the trauma victims quickly and to transport them, equally rapidly, to a nearby centre of medical excellence. The other, perhaps more controversial, concept is one of "stay and play". If the patient is critically injured and evacuation time is likely to be long or may be delayed by entrapment or for logistic reasons, it is suggested that advanced trauma life support skills be taken to the incident. In this way, medical personnel with the appropriate equipment may be able to resuscitate and stabilise casualties who might otherwise die before arrival at hospital.[12]

There can be no authoritative advice to cover all occasions. Often, decisions can be made only at the accident scene and must, by necessity, take into account a wide range of factors such as the location of the incident, the number of casualties, and the distance and time to the most appropriate medical facility.[15] The helicopter offers great advantages over road transport, especially in being able to approach incidents where access is difficult or where roads may not even exist. Confined spaces (particularly in urban areas) are not necessarily a problem and, when time is of the essence, patients can be delivered to the most appropriate hospital for their injuries, which may not necessarily be the nearest one. The helicopter therefore becomes not just a means of transportation but also an airborne intensive care unit, making immediate medical care as immediate as it can be, and thereby diminishing the duration of the therapeutic vacuum. The result is not simply a reduction in mortality, but also of disability, with recovery promoted by effective shortening of time in hospital and time before return to useful work.[16]

Fixed wing aircraft

Although less expensive to operate than helicopters, fixed wing aircraft suffer from the single major disadvantage of requiring large expanses of open flat terrain to be able to collect and deliver their human cargo. Because hospitals are rarely conveniently located near airports, this inevitably necessitates ground transfers at either end of the flight and fixed wing aircraft are therefore only occasionally used in the primary response role, and then usually only when distances are great.

With increasing affluence, more leisure time and the introduction of relatively inexpensive and easily accessible means of travel, tourism has expanded dramatically in recent years: so too has the need to repatriate those unfortunates who have been injured or who have fallen ill many miles from home. International travel is now an unexceptional experience, and often little thought is given by travellers to the potential health problems of their destination.[17] Although many will consider vaccination against low risk endemic infectious diseases, they fail to appreciate such factors as local hygiene practices, climate, food, the risks of accidental injury, and possible limitations of any medical facilities. In 1991, more than 30 000 British travellers abroad requested some form of medical assistance by means of travel insurance. One company alone repatriated over 2000 patients; just under half requiring either a medical or nursing escort. It has been calculated that one in 500 travellers requests some form of help and one in 10 000 requires emergency repatriation.[18]

In this repatriation role, different aircraft types are used for different mission assignments. Ambulant patients may travel in conventional passenger carrying aircraft and may need only some form of medical supervision, with the provision of emergency drugs and equipment, for the possibility of any untoward problem occurring during the transfer (see chapter 3). These patients may require wheelchair transportation within the chaotic and demanding confines of a busy airport terminal with perhaps facilitated transit through the essential arrival and departure formalities, but they might otherwise be treated like any other passenger.

Patients with minor disability or encumbrance might be offered seating with more leg room (perhaps in upper class), although safety regulations stipulate that disabled passengers must not sit directly next to emergency exits.[19] An alternative might be to allocate two seats to allow more lateral space. Stretchers can be carried on many aircraft types, but usually necessitate the allocation of a block of nine conventional seats. The stretcher frame is bolted securely to the lower half of the folded seats in a single column of three and the remaining seats are used to hold medical equipment and for the medical escort's seating. Large aircraft dedicated to the air ambulance role (almost exclusively military) are usually converted so that the passenger seats are replaced by frames that can carry multiple stretchers stacked on top of each other. The design and comfort of these conversions depend on the role of the aircraft. Large tactical aircraft (such as the Lockheed C130 Hercules) trade creature comforts for robustness, whereas those used in the strategic role (such as the Lockheed TriStar) are faster, less noisy, and will maintain the passenger cabin decor and fit when converted to carry stretchers.

Critically ill patients are difficult to manage on conventional passenger carrying aircraft, and airline medical authorities may refuse medical clearance for some types of patient (see chapter 3). These aircraft are not designed to carry the medical equipment that is so often needed in the care of the seriously ill and, despite screening, it is almost impossible to maintain privacy from the inquisitive eyes of other passengers. Whenever possible, then, small dedicated air ambulance aircraft are used to transport those in need of intensive therapy, and those who might otherwise be refused carriage by the airlines. When distances are short, piston or turboprop aircraft are used. Many of these aircraft are unpressurised and it may be necessary to consider the patient's requirements for inflight oxygen. Over greater distances, faster jet aircraft are used. These are invariably pressurised, but care must be taken in establishing the optimum pressure schedule for those whose oxygen carrying capability is impaired (see chapter 3). The final decision on the aircraft type best suited to any individual medical transfer is a fine balance, based on speed, range, cabin size, internal fit and cost.

The cost of a dedicated aeromedical flight depends very much on the aircraft type, destination and on the medical requirements in transit. For example, to retrieve a seriously ill patient from Spain and deliver him to a hospital in the United Kingdom is unlikely to cost less than £7000. This expense is out of the reach of the average traveller, and health insurance is essential. Great care must be taken, however, in choosing the right medical cover (especially if adventurous sports are anticipated or manual work is planned), and all pre-existing illness must be declared. Potentially expensive disappointment can occur if cover is withdrawn after the event because the illness or injury is outside of the terms of the original agreement. Although reciprocal health services are available within the European Community (on production of a valid form E111), this entitlement covers only the cost of emergency treatment, and does not extend to the expense of repatriation.

Anticipating potential problems

There are few clinical reasons for refusal of aeromedical transportation, and none is absolute. However, a knowledge and understanding of the physical, physiological and psychological constraints imposed by the flight environment will allow anticipation, and therefore prevention, of clinical problems that may occur in flight or at any other stage of the transfer. The upper troposphere is a hostile place. As air pressure declines, less oxygen is available for cellular metabolism and gases trapped within body cavities will expand. There may be problems with motion sickness, vibration, noise, cold or humidity, not to mention the psychological terror felt by someone who can imagine nothing worse than being locked in a metal tube flying at 805 kph (500 mph) at an altitude of 10 670 m (35 000 ft). These problems are described in chapters 1, 3, and 5.

In the confines of an aircraft, the major functional disadvantage to the practice of medicine is one of space. A patient (and possibly relatives) plus flight crew and medical team, with their equipment and baggage, soon consume all available space within the cabin. Simply opening an equipment box or bag may prove difficult, and major medical interventions may be almost impossible. Prior planning and positioning of essential equipment may alleviate some potential problems, but there is no sbustitute for frequent practice and training in the aircraft cabin itself (or a cabin space mockup).

Also, when considering the effects on the patient of a long distance transfer, awareness of (and planning for) logistic factors such as the duration of out-of-hospital time, ground transfers, airport formalities, inflight facilities/equipment/skills, airborne sector times, time zone changes, stopovers, changes of aircraft, medical facilities at each stage, and the actual time of arrival at the destination facility, is absolutely vital. In addition, consideration must be given to the provision and timing of feeding and medications in transit, and to the availability of suitable clothing or protection when travelling between one climate and another. This list is not exhaustive and does not include such nonmedical but essential issues such as the availability of emergency funds in suitable currencies, passports, visas and documentation for the import/export of controlled drugs.

The overall aim is to transfer the patient safely from point of origin to destination, causing no further harm. If useful treatment can be started or continued, then so much the better. Essentially, care in the air should not fall short of that which can be found on the ground. This is a tall order when consideration is given to the constraints already listed, but its achievement can be helped by ensuring that adequate medical equipment and medications are available during transit, that members of the flight medical team are thoroughly familiar with their usage, and that they have the knowledge and skills to deal with both the predictable and the unexpected.

Equipment

Recent years have seen the design and modification of portable equipment ideally suited to use in aircraft. Such equipment must be compact, lightweight and rugged enough to withstand the stresses of acceleration, vibration, and the possibility of rapid decompression. Those items which are electrically powered must be compatible with aircaft supplies and should be capable of independent battery operation when disconnected from the aircraft. The battery life should be adequate for the duration of the entire transit, with sufficient reserves for unexpected delays and diversions. Similarly, oxygen powered machines must have adequate reserves which will not erode those necessary for the patient's own respiratory requirements.

The items of equipment to be carried will, naturally, depend both on the role of the aircraft and on the specific problems of the patient(s) being escorted. The equipment carried can be grouped according to type: in addition to obvious diagnostic and therapeutic medical machinery and matériel, items needed may include ambulance equipment (stretchers, splints, blankets, extrication and immobilisation devices, et cetera), personal safety and rescue items (helmets, gloves, protective clothing, metal cutters, et cetera) and communication devices (radio transmitters and mobile telephones). For example, in the EMS role, the minimum diagnostic and therapeutic equipment carried should include an electrocardiogram monitor, defibrillator, pulse oximeter, noninvasive blood pressure monitor, suction aspirator, mechanical ventilator, and all equipment necessary to perform safely any of the procedures recommended in the advanced cardiac life support and the advanced trauma life support protocols appropriate to the prehospital environment.[20-22] Table 4.3 lists items of equipment which are susceptible to gaseous expansion during flight.

Several attempts to standardise aeromedical equipment scales have been made in the recent past,[23-25] but the Commission Européenne de Normalisation, although recently embarked on the task of standardising land ambulance equipment throughout Europe, has deferred addressing the complexities of air ambulance equipment because of the wide diversity of aircraft types and missions.[26] Whatever equipment is carried, it must be properly maintained under a servicing schedule which takes account of the rigours imposed by the aeromedical environment. Equipment and

---

TABLE 4.3—Equipment susceptible to gaseous expansion

- Sphygmomanometer cuffs
- Glass intravenous fluid bottles
- Pressure bags
- Intravenous administration sets
- Pressurised antishock garments
- Chest drains
- Nasogastric tubes and other closed drains
- Endotracheal tube cuffs
- Catheter balloons
- Air splints

---

medical matériel (especially disposable items and those requiring cleaning or sterilisation) must be thoroughly checked before and on completion of each assignment and should be safely fitted or stowed in the aircraft during flight, and in the corresponding land ambulance during any associated ground transfer.

Some dedicated aircraft will have permanent, fixed equipment. Such equipment may prove hazardous in terms of spurious electromagnetic fields (which may interfere with radio communications and navigation avionics), and may present a loose object hazard risk during impact or emergency landings, so each item must be checked, tested and cleared for use by the relevant national aviation authority. Mobile equipment must also be cleared, although it is understood that some items may be required at short notice and a commonsense attitude must prevail, with close liaison between medical and flight crews to ensure safe operation.

Training

In terms of flight medical personnel, several countries have broached the concept of standardisation of training and experience requirements.[23-25] Once again, however, there is a dilemma caused by the wide variation in types of missions undertaken by aeromedical personnel. Certainly it is essential for the medical crew to have a thorough understanding of the safety aspects of the aircraft in which they are flying, including the use of all cabin safety equipment during inflight emergencies. Other aviation related aspects are taught to personnel in some EMS systems, and depend on the extent of aircrew workload expected of the medical crewperson. Subjects such as navigation, meteorology, radio procedures and principles of flight are, for example, more relevant to the paramedic working full time on an EMS helicopter or on search and rescue duties than to the flight nurse who repatriates rehabilitated patients on large passenger carrying aircraft only a few times a month.

Similarly, medical skills will be dependent on role and assignment. All medical personnel must be thoroughly familiar with advanced cardiac life support and advanced trauma life support procedures, and should preferably have experience in anaesthesiology, intensive care or emergency medicine, in addition to a working knowledge of the principles of aviation physiology. Similar exposure to resuscitation skills is required by paramedics and nurses who are assigned to flight duties. Over and above these basic requirements, individual patients may demand specific skills (and equipment) which must be available when required: for example neonates, psychiatric patients, and those with spinal injuries or burns. Although medical personnel work largely unsupervised in the aeromedical role, they are not excused from the normal responsibilities of their profession; that is, from their duties with regard to standards of care, confidentiality and documentation.

Aircrew must also be highly trained and experienced, especially those EMS pilots who frequently operate from confined spaces under difficult conditions. In addition to their flying skills, they must have enough basic medical training to understand the pathophysiology of serious illness and multiple trauma, and the effects of transportation. Because aircrew are often called upon to assist the medical team at the accident scene, or during the embarkation of patients, it is also essential that they have an absolute familiarity with the medical equipment carried, and with the procedures for safe loading and unloading of patients.

The way ahead

The carriage of patients by air has progressed and developed rapidly during the latter part of the twentieth century. As the new millennium approaches, further advancement is inevitable. Bigger aircraft will fly faster, perhaps higher, and certainly for a longer time, making even more destinations accessible on single sector passages, and to more potential travellers than ever. Communications and telemetry may well allow closer supervision of aeromedical escorts in transit, and the use of computerised diagnostics (such as the automatic defibrillator) and new dry-reagent biochemical tests (like Clinistix) will make treatment decisions more reliable. Equipment is becoming increasingly miniaturised, reliable and affordable. Small, dependable capnographs are now being introduced as a means of detecting misplacement of endotracheal tubes,[27] and other noninvasive monitoring techniques (for example, of cerebral blood flow and cardiac output) are in the early stages of investigation.[28,29]

In the field of training, emergency medical care has recently taken centre stage as a wider realisation dawns that trauma is still the "neglected disease" and remains the most common killer of the young,[9,30] and that acute cardiovascular disease is a frequent cause of death in the middle aged.[31] The advent of new training courses with subsequent recognition by examination has been universally welcomed. A new awareness exists that every medical practitioner must be able to manage the essential initial stages of resuscitation: but training is of little value without ongoing research and development of new ideas. As international travel continues to increase, and growth of the aeromedical industry follows, the application of new ideas and technologies is likely to result in major innovations in the logistics of patient carriage by air, and in the development of proper integration of transport systems within the total emergency medical care organisation.

1 Meier DR, Samper ER. Evolution of civil aeromedical helicopter evaucation. *South Med J* 1989; **82**: 885–91.
2 Cook JL. *Dust off*. New York: Rufus, 1988.
3 Trunkey D. Towards optimal trauma care. *Arch Emerg Med* 1985; **2**: 181–95.
4 Liskiewicz WJ. An evaluation of the Royal Air Force helicopter search and rescue service in Britain with reference to Royal Air Force Valley 1980–1989. *J R Soc Med* 1992; **85**: 727–9.
5 Nicholson PJ. The helicopter in the immediate care environment. *J Br Assoc Immed Care* 1988; **11**: 54–7.
6 Dalling J. It's all go on the Sea King. *RAF News* 1992: **Oct 30.**
7 Martin TE. Al Jubail—an aeromedical staging facility during the Gulf conflict. *J R Soc Med* 1992; **85**: 32–6.
8 *Flight deck, Falklands edition*. London: Ministry of Defence, 1982.
9 National Academy of Sciences, National Research Council. *Accidental death and disability, the neglected disease of modern society*. Washington DC: US Government Printing Office, 1966.
10 Day D. Value of medical helicopter programs debated as the number of helicopter accidents increases. *Emerg Med Amb Care News* 1987; **9**: 1.
11 Ramage C, Kee S, Bristow A. Interhospital transfer of the critically ill by helicopter. *Br J Hosp Med* 1990; **43**: 147.
12 Coats TJ, Wilson AW. Utilization of the Helicopter Emergency Medical Service. *J R Soc Med* 1992; **85**: 725–6.
13 Sellwood NH, Westaway P. The Cornwall air ambulance. *J Br Assoc Immed Care* 1988; **11**: 59–63.
14 Wilson A, Cross F. Helicopters. *J R Soc Med* 1992; **85**: 1–2.
15 Martin TE. Resolving the casualty evacuation conflict. *Injury* 1993 **24**: 514–16.
16 Schwartz RJ, Jacobs LM, Yaezel D. Impact of pre-trauma centre care on length of stay and hospital charges. *J Trauma* 1989; **29**: 1611–17.
17 Porter JDH, Stanwell-Smith R, Lea G. Travelling hopefully, returning ill. *BMJ* 1992; **304**: 1323–4.
18 Fairhurst RJ. Health insurance for international travel. In: Dawood R, ed. *Travellers' health*, 3rd edn. Oxford: Oxford University Press, 1992: 371–5.
19 Green RL, Mooney SE. Carriage of invalid passengers by civil airlines. In: Ernsting J, King PF, eds. *Aviation medicine*. London: Butterworths, 1988.
20 *Textbook of advanced cardiac life support*. Dallas: American Heart Association, 1987.
21 *Advanced trauma life support course*. Chicago: Committee on Trauma, American College of Surgeons, 1988.
22 ALS Working Party of the ERC. Guidelines for advanced cardiac life support. *Resuscitation* 1992; **24**: 111–21.
23 US Department of Trade National Highway Traffic Safety Administration and American Medical Association Commission on Emergency Medical Services. *Air Ambulance Guidelines*, 1986.

24 Working Party Report. Medical helicopter systems—recommended minimum standards for patient management. *J R Soc Med* 1991; **84:** 242–4.
25 Working Party Report. Recommended standards for UK fixed wing medical air transport systems and for patient management during transfer by fixed wing aircraft. *J R Soc Med* 1992; **85:** 767–71.
26 Ward M. European standardisation of ambulance equipment. *J Br Assoc Immed Care* 1993; **16:** 2.
27 Anonymous. Mini-Cap III—CO_2 monitor. *J Br Assoc Immed Care* 1991; **14:** 80.
28 Glaister DH, Martin TE. The application of near-infrared spectroscopy to aviation medicine research. *Aviat Space Environ Med* 1991; **62:** 477.
29 World MJ. Estimation of cardiac output by bioimpedance cardiography. *J R Army Med Corps* 1990; **136:** 92–9.
30 World Health Organization. *World health statistics annual.* Geneva: WHO, 1989.
31 Hampton J. Prognosis in ischaemic heart disease. *Med Int* 1989; **68:** 2818–23.

5
Problems of altitude

He rode upon the cherubims, and did fly: he came flying upon the wings of the wind.[1]

Concorde commonly cruises at altitudes of 15 240–18 288 m (50 000–60 000 ft) where, if unprotected, its occupants would be unconscious within 15 s and dead 4–6 min later from lack of oxygen.[2] Even at the more usual cruising altitudes of commercial aircraft—9144–12 192 m (30 000–40 000 ft)—unprotected passengers and crew would rapidly succumb. Of course this does not happen, thanks to the protection of the aircraft pressure cabin. The wellbeing of the air traveller within this artificial environment is, however, always threatened by the problems of altitude extending beyond lack of oxygen to decompression illness, cold, and simple pressure effects.

Physics of the atmosphere

Ascent to altitude is associated with a fall in air pressure paralleled by decreases in density and temperature. Thus at 5486 m (18 000 ft) atmospheric pressure is half its value at sea level and the ambient temperature is about $-20°C$ (fig 5.1). The fall in total atmospheric pressure and the consequent reduction in the partial pressure of oxygen (Po_2) poses the greatest single threat to anyone who flies: hypoxia. Fortunately, the relationship between oxygen saturation of haemoglobin and oxygen tension, reflected in the shape of the oxygen dissociation curve, minimises the effect. The plateau represents an inbuilt reserve, which is exploited by aircraft designers, and provides protection against hypoxia up to an altitude of 3048 m (10 000 ft) (fig 5.2). Ascent to this altitude produces a fall in alveolar Po_2 from the normal 13·7 kPa (103 mmHg) to 8·0 kPa (60 mmHg) but only a slight fall in percentage saturation of haemoglobin with oxygen. As altitude

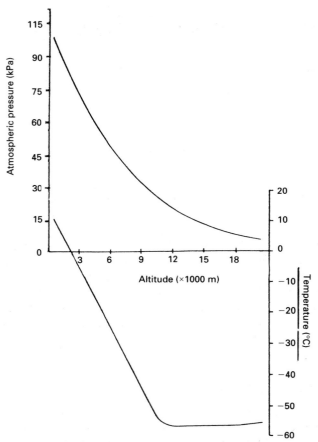

FIG 5.1—Relations between altitude and pressure and altitude and temperature. (100 mmHg ≃ 13·3 kPa; 5000 ft ≃ 1500 m).

progressively rises above 3048 m (10 000 ft) the percentage saturation of haemoglobin falls precipitously and hypoxia is the result.

Cabin pressurisation and decompression

Commercial aircraft cabins are pressurised to below 3048 m (10 000 ft)—and usually to 1525–2134 m (5000–7000 ft)—both as a safety margin for passengers and because psychomotor performance at novel tasks, which is of relevance to aircrew, deteriorates at

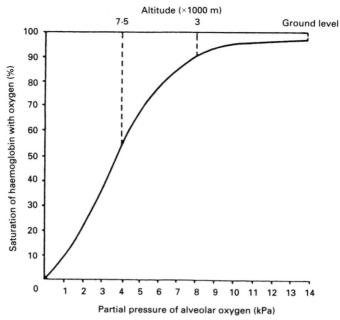

FIG 5.2—Relation between partial pressure of alveolar oxygen, percentage saturation of haemoglobin with oxygen, and altitude. (1 kPa $\simeq$ 8 mmHg; 5000 ft $\simeq$ 1500 m.)

altitudes above about 2438 m (8000 ft).[3] Pressurisation to sea level, although ideal, is not cost effective.

Aircraft maintain a positive ambient pressure within their cabins by drawing in external air and delivering it, compressed, to the cabin. The outflow of cabin air is then controlled so as to maintain the required pressure differential. The through flow also ventilates the cabin and provides a means by which the ambient temperature may be controlled. As long as the pressurisation system and the aircraft remain intact, protection is provided at normal operating altitudes. In practice the degree of pressurisation increases linearly with, but at a slower rate than, actual altitude, from ground level to a high maximum differential pressure (fig 5.3). Thereafter, cabin altitude increases at the same rate as aircraft altitude along a line determined by the pressure characteristics of the hull: the maximum differential pressure line.

The problems of altitude become manifest if and when cabin pressurisation fails. Such failures still occur in both civil and

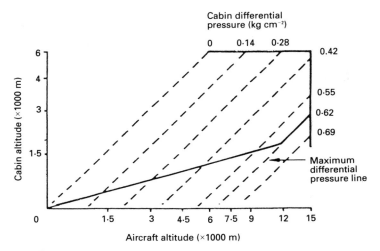

FIG 5.3—Typical passenger aircraft pressurisation profile. In this example the maximum differential pressure line is reached when the aircraft altitude is 12 040 m (39 500 ft) and cabin altitude is 1829 m (6000 ft). (1 lb in^{-2} $\simeq 0.06$ kg cm^{-2}; 5000 ft $\simeq 1500$ m.)

military aircraft, large and small.[4-6] In the case of a slow loss of pressure—for example, as a result of malfunction of a control system—the cabin altitude will increase slowly; this is usually rapidly recognised and dealt with by the crew. The main danger is hypoxia in susceptible subjects. Effects are more dramatic when a rapid decompression occurs—for example, when a window is lost or when the pressure hull is ruptured. The latter may happen as a result of terrorist action, as in the Lockerbie disaster, or as a consequence of metal fatigue, as in the loss of most of the forward cabin structure of the Aloha Airlines aircraft in April 1988. In these cases there is a massive movement of air out through the defect, which will carry with it any loose articles and even passengers close to the breach who are not wearing their seat belts.[4] The air movement creates considerable noise and the sudden cooling causes condensation and misting, thus making both communication and vision difficult. These initial events are rapidly succeeded by the problems of hypoxia, perhaps complicated by cold injury (frostbite and frostnip), and decompression illness. The rate, duration, and effects of rapid decompression depend on the external and cabin altitudes at the moment of decompression, the volume of the cabin, and the size of the defect.

61

Combat aircraft are pressurised to a lesser degree so as to achieve a lower structural weight, and to improve the power:weight ratio. In addition, the risk of sudden loss of cabin pressure in these aircraft is increased as a result of enemy action. The degree of pressurisation depends on actual altitude, as in commercial aircraft. The oxygen deficit when cabin altitudes exceed 3048 m (10 000 ft) in military aircraft is compensated for by oxygen enrichment of the inspired air as altitude increases, until at about 9144 m (30 000 ft) 100% oxygen is being delivered. The supply, conventionally from a gaseous or liquid oxygen source but occasionally from a molecular sieve oxygen concentrator,[7] is fed individually to each crew member through a demand regulator and oronasal mask.

Hypoxia

Physiological factors

The earliest feature of acute hypobaric hypoxia is often a subtle personality change perhaps coupled with euphoria, lack of judgement, loss of short term memory, and mental incoordination. This combination is not unpleasant and resembles the early stages of alcoholic intoxication, but its insidiousness is of the greatest danger to the victim.[5] In a crew member it may be disastrous because he or she may well be unaware of failing performance. Subsequent features reflect the stimulation of cardiovascular and respiratory compensatory mechanisms. In moderate hypoxia—for example when air breathing at 7620 m (25 000 ft)[6]—cardiac output and heart rate are increased but overall peripheral resistance is reduced, so that mean arterial blood pressure is unchanged. Cerebral blood flow is increased, although the degree of increase is modified by the magnitude of coexisting hypocapnia which results from increased respiratory minute volume. Thus cerebral and cardiac perfusion are increased at the expense of less vital organs. Muscular incoordination develops—including slurred speech—and this, together with loss of touch sensation, may prevent the victim from taking effective remedial action. The special senses are also affected; classically, tunnelling of vision occurs, although nonspecific visual symptoms are more common. Loss of auditory acuity is a late feature, however, and even then is not pronounced. Respiration increases under the hypoxic drive to help alleviate cerebral hypoxia but is ineffective, and the symptoms and signs of hyperventilation develop alongside those of hypoxia. Hyperventilation is a normal response to a fall in alveolar Po_2 to below 7·3–8·0 kPa (55–60 mmHg) and may be the dominant clinical feature. Lightheadedness, feelings of unreality and anxiety, paraesthesiae, visual disturbances—for example blurring and scotomata—and palpitations are common in people exposed suddenly to altitudes of 7620 m (25 000 ft).

The features of hypoxia vary between subjects and the rate at which they develop depends on the severity of the hypoxic insult. Thus most of the changes described occur within 3–5 min of sudden exposure to an altitude of 7620 m (25 000 ft) (by which time alveolar $Po_2 = 4·0$ kPa (30 mmHg) and alveolar $Pco_2 = 2·9$ kPa (22 mmHg)),[6] but above 13 716 m (45 000 ft) unconsciousness, often preceded by convulsions, supervenes within 15–20 s.

The treatment of hypobaric hypoxia is with oxygen. In passenger aircraft, oxygen is delivered through automatic dropdown sets whenever the cabin altitude exceeds a certain level, usually 3658–4267 m (12 000–14 000 ft). Each set has a mask attached which should be placed over the face immediately. In many systems the action of pulling the mask, with its delivery tube attached, on to the face initiates the flow of oxygen, but even this simple manoeuvre may be beyond the ability of passengers exposed to rapid decompression at high altitude.[4,8] Manipulating equipment may be further complicated if the stricken aircraft subsequently descends rapidly, and the passengers are flexed forward in their seats. Seats facing backwards would prevent such flexing and so make the oxygen mask easier to use.[9] The flight deck crew are equipped with more elaborate oxygen systems—similar to those in military aircraft—to enable them to accomplish, unimpaired, a rapid descent to a safe altitude of less than 3048 m (10 000 ft). The cabin staff also have portable oxygen sets for their own use while helping passengers.

A degree of hypoxia will develop in all occupants of an aircraft when breathing air at altitudes above 3048 m (10 000 ft). Some people may, however, become hypoxic below this altitude and will require therapeutic oxygen in the aircraft. Oxygen in these circumstances may be given through the passenger's own automatic set or from a portable emergency supply.

Occasionally symptoms and signs worsen transiently when oxygen is restored to a hypoxic patient. This *oxygen paradox* probably results from a combination of a reflex peripheral arteriolar vasodilatation, with consequent hypotension, and a persistent cerebral vasoconstriction due to the hypocapnia associated with hypoxia.[6] The phenomenon is usually mild and lasts for 15–60 s, after which recovery is rapid provided that oxygen administration is maintained. On rare occasions, however, the paradox may produce convulsions and loss of consciousness.

Medical factors (see also chapter 3)

Many factors may cause one person to be more susceptible to lack of oxygen than another: ill health, especially cardiovascular and respiratory disorders, may lead to problems; alcohol and other drugs, particularly proprietary cold cures (and especially those containing antihistamines), may potentiate the lack of oxygen; and carbon monoxide preferentially displaces oxygen from the haemoglobin molecule so that smoking may raise carboxyhaemoglobin concentrations sufficiently to reduce the inbuilt reserve, despite enzymic and haematological compensatory mechanisms. In addition, the interaction of carbon monoxide with haemoglobin shifts the oxygen dissociation curve to the left, further reducing the amount of oxygen available for release to the tissues.[10] Thus a heavy smoker may already be at an equivalent altitude of several thousand feet while walking to the aircraft. Finally, any condition that increases oxygen requirements, such as exercise or cold, will reduce tolerance to hypoxia.

Hyperventilation

Hypoxia is not the only cause of hyperventilation in flight, but it is the most important and difficult aspect of the differential diagnosis of hyperventilation. Causes include other environmental stresses, such as whole body vibration in air turbulence, motion sickness, and high ambient temperatures. The most common cause, however, is anxiety or emotional stress. A large proportion of aircrew under training hyperventilate,[11] as do experienced aircrew, especially when confronted with an unusual or severe mental stress such as inflight emergency. Passengers who are inexperienced air travellers are often affected. The symptoms and signs of hyperventilation (as described above) are all attributable to the resulting hypocapnia.[12] Unconsciousness or even tetany are rare occurrences. The usual clinical picture is an increasingly anxious passenger, with early symptoms, requiring help. The simple but effective technique of rebreathing expired air is the treatment of choice, together with a logical explanation of events and firm instructions to breathe more slowly. Caution in the use of the classic method of rebreathing from a paper bag has recently been advised on the grounds that it may exacerbate hypoxia to a significant extent at cabin altitudes.[13] Passengers who habitually hyperventilate may need sedation before the flight; experience and training will reduce the likelihood of hyperventilation among crew members.

Despite the fact that hyperventilation is probably more common than hypoxia during flight, aircrew must assume that any suspicious symptoms or signs are due to hypoxia whenever the cabin altitude exceeds 3048 m (10 000 ft) and not to hyperventilation from another cause. They must also take appropriate remedial action. The importance of the similarities between hyperventilation due to hypoxia and hyperventilation alone, and the possibly fatal implications of misdiagnosis, should be emphasised during training.

Subatmospheric (aviator's) decompression sickness (dysbarism)

Rapid ascent to altitude also carries with it the threat of decompression sickness, another potentially fatal condition. Although the precise mechanism in humans has never been unequivocally determined, decompression sickness almost certainly results from supersaturation of body tissues with nitrogen as ambient pressure falls, which leads to bubbles developing in the blood and tissues.[14] This supersaturation is a consequence of the relatively poor solubility of nitrogen in the blood, so that the rate of fall of the partial pressure of nitrogen in the tissues lags behind that of the absolute pressure on ascent to altitude. The tendency for bubbles to form around nuclei, such as vessel wall irregularities, is greater as the difference between the two pressures increases. Once established the bubbles grow in size and may be carried by the circulation to other parts of the body where they produce the various clinical manifestations of the condition.

Clinical features

The "bends"—Joint pain is the most common symptom of aviator's (and diver's) decompression sickness, and is seen in about

65

74% of cases after exposure to 8534 m (28 600 ft) for 2 hours.[15] The pain is probably due to extravascular bubble formation around and within affected joints and usually develops in a single large joint— the knee, the shoulder, the elbow, or the wrist, in that order of frequency. A mild ache, characteristically made worse by movement, progresses to a severe pain that radiates along the affected limb.

The "creeps"—Dermal manifestations are seen infrequently (in about 7%) and are probably the result of bubbles being carried to the skin from other sites. Formication and paraesthesiae may be accompanied by localised rashes, urticaria, and skin mottling. The significance of the creeps is that they may be indicative of more serious underlying problems.

The "chokes"—Although also infrequent (about 5%), respiratory symptoms are serious features which lead to collapse if untreated. They are probably due to a reflex response to the presence of bubbles within the pulmonary microcirculation. Feelings of chest constriction and retrosternal pain are associated with coughing, which may become paroxysmal when an attempt is made to take a deep breath.

The "staggers"—Neurological manifestations are rare (about 1%) and result from evolved gas bubble embolism within the central nervous system. A variety of features is involved, including anaesthesia, paralysis, and convulsions. Visual disturbances (about 2%) usually consist of blurred vision, scotomas, or hemianopia. In an appreciable number of neurological cases (about 9%) the victim may develop malaise, anxiety, and a reduced level of consciousness, without other symptoms and signs (a primary collapse) or with them (a secondary collapse). This syndrome of cerebral decompression sickness may progress to one of profound shock.

A second neurological syndrome—arterial gas embolism—may very rarely be associated with rapid decompression to high altitude (although it is more common in the *hyper*baric environment). In this condition, overinflation of pulmonary tissue results in rupture of alveoli and escape of gas directly into the arterial circulation. Subsequent embolisation to the brain can produce a clinical picture very similar to cerebral decompression sickness, and it is because of this similarity that the global term decompression *illness* has recently been recommended as a replacement for the more familiar decompression *sickness*.[16] Amplification of the title by an evolutionary term (such as static, relapsing, or progressive) and a manifestation term (such as cutaneous, neurological, limb pain, or multisystem) has also been recommended as a means of overcoming the confusion which surrounds the many classifications used at present, and of allowing greater collaboration and comparison between different reporting centres.

Treatment

Victims of aviator's decompression sickness require immediate recompression. Most recover immediately or very soon after descent to ground level, and usually well before. The patient should be given 100% oxygen, if available, during the descent and kept warm and still. In addition, local pressure applied to an affected joint usually relieves the pain. Persistent and severe cases may need hyperbaric treatment after landing, and the ground emergency services should be alerted to this possibility during descent. Occasionally, usually following exposure to altitudes greater than 8534 m (28 000 ft), during which severe symptoms of decompression may[15] or may not[17] have developed, the symptoms may become worse on landing. The cause is probably widespread gas bubble embolism and, if coma follows the profound cardiovascular and neurological collapse, recovery without treatment is rare. Arterial gas embolism is very serious and requires immediate recompression.

Predisposing factors

Fortunately, subatmospheric decompression sickness is not common. It is almost unknown in healthy subjects at altitudes of less than 5486 m (18 000 ft) (but see below) and is rare between 5486 and 7620 m (18 000–25 000 ft). Above this level decompression sickness occurs with increasing frequency and severity with increasing altitude.[15] Thus (together with hypoxia and the problems of cold injury) it is a distinct hazard after loss of cabin pressure at normal cruising altitudes and has claimed at least one life in the recent past.[18] With the ever greater numbers of general aviation (private) aircraft flying, unpressurised, to altitudes of 5486 m (18 000 ft) and above, decompression sickness may be an increasing risk for these aviators.[19]

Decompression sickness rarely develops until at least 5 min—and more usually 20–60 min—have passed at altitude, by which time descent should have begun. Various factors may decrease tolerance to decompression sickness so that it may develop at altitudes below 5486 m (18 000 ft) and occasionally below 3048 m (10 000 ft): thus ill health, drugs, alcohol, exercise, cold, and hypoxia all increase the possibility of decompression sickness, as do age (susceptibility is increased ninefold between 17–20 and 27–29 years), obesity (adipose tissue has a high content of dissolved nitrogen and relatively poor blood supply), and previous exposure to decompression. Instances of the last may occur after several unpressurised flights in rapid succession—for example parachute training at high altitudes—or, or more subtly, subaqua diving,[20] during which nitrogen is compressed into the tissues. Although some of this nitrogen will evolve into gas during ascent (decompression) to the water's surface, more than usual will be present to form more gas bubbles if an ascent to altitude is undertaken shortly afterwards.

Finally, an as yet unexplained true individual susceptibility to decompression sickness does seem to occur.

There is a bewildering number of guidelines about flying after diving for the recreational diver: for example, there are 30 published sets of recommendations for those who wish to fly after diving within standard air tables; five more for saturation divers; and a further 12 to guide those concerned with the inflight management of decompression illness or with flying after hyperbaric therapy.[21] It is wise to select a single reference and in the United Kingdom the *Royal Navy Diving Manual*, although aimed primarily at service divers, is well known and authoritative:[22] article 5122 of the manual provides simple advice on the minimum intervals between diving and flying, for dives without or with stops (see table 5.1), and article 5121 gives advice for those who intend flying after diving at altitude (for example in mountain lakes). In the United States, very similar guidelines are recommended by the Federal Aviation Administration and the Undersea and Hyperbaric Medicine Society.[23] More stringent regulations apply to aircrew who may have participated in sports diving.

Pressure changes in gas containing cavities

Because the body temperature is constant any gas within closed or semiclosed cavities will essentially obey Boyle's law on ascent to altitude; for example, any such gas will have doubled in volume—if it is free to expand—at 5486 m (18 000 ft), where atmospheric

TABLE 5.1—Flying after diving: recommended time intervals*

Type of dive	Time interval between diving and flying (hours)	Approximate maximum altitude (or effective altitude in pressurised aircraft) (m (ft))
Without stops	≤ 1	300 (1000)†
	1–2	1500 (5000)
	> 2	Unlimited flying in commercial aircraft (normally no more than an effective 2400 m (8000 ft) above sea level)
With stops	≤ 4	300 (1000)†
	4–8	1500 (5000)
	8–24	5000 (16 500)
	> 24	Unlimited

*After Ministry of Defence.[22]
†For example helicopters

pressure is half that at sea level. The lungs, the teeth, the gut, the middle ear, and the sinuses may all be affected.

Problems on ascent

Expansion of gas in the lungs does not usually present a hazard because excess gas is easily vented by the trachea. The lungs are extremely unlikely to be damaged unless a rapid decompression of catastrophic magnitude occurs and the glottis is closed at the moment of decompression.

Pain in a tooth on ascent (aerodontalgia) may occur but is uncommon. Although its precise cause is disputed, aerodontalgia arises when overt or covert dental disorders already exist, and it may be that the change in atmospheric pressure irritates the circulation in a diseased pulp. Alternatively, the relative increase in pressure within a closed air space beneath a dental filling or carious deposit may cause pain by a neural or vascular mechanism. Whatever the cause, this condition is one reason why aircrew should receive regular dental inspections because it does not occur in healthy or correctly restored teeth.[24]

Expansion of gas in the small intestine can cause severe pain and subsequent vasovagal syncope. This is unlikely during a slow ascent to low cabin altitudes in passenger aircraft but may occur during rapid decompression undertaken for training purposes and may also follow rapid loss of cabin pressure at high altitude. In

69

normal circumstances passengers may notice slight abdominal distension, which may be enough to affect the well being of travellers with cardiovascular or respiratory disorders. Intestinal expansion is aggravated by foods and drinks which produce gas such as beans, curries, brassicas, and alcohol. Gas in the stomach or large intestine can easily be released and does not cause problems.

Problems on descent

Gas expanding in the middle ear cavity vents through the eustachian tube on ascent and only rarely causes any discomfort in the eardrum—the ears merely "pop". Symptoms arise on descent because air cannot pass back up the tube. Pain, which begins as a feeling of increasing pressure on the tympanic membrane, quickly becomes severe and progressive unless the eustachian tube is able to open and equalise pressure between the middle ear and the atmosphere. In most people this may be achieved by swallowing, yawning, or moving the lower jaw from side to side, but others have to perform a deliberate manoeuvre to open the tube by raising the pressure in the nasopharynx.[25] The most useful of these techniques is the frenzel manoeuvre, in which the mouth, nostrils, and epiglottis are closed and air in the nasopharynx is compressed by the action of the muscles of the mouth and tongue. This technique generates higher nasopharyngeal pressures than the valsalva manoeuvre and opens the eustachian tube at lower pressures.[26] The valsalva manoeuvre consists of a forced expiration through an open glottis while the mouth is shut and the nostrils occluded. The increase in intrathoracic pressure is transmitted to the nasopharynx and hence to the eustachian tubes. The rise in intrathoracic pressure is a disadvantage, however, because it impedes venous return to the heart and may even induce syncope. In a third eponymous technique, the toynbee manoeuvre, pharyngeal pressure is raised by swallowing while the mouth is closed and the nostrils occluded.

Unfortunately, the acute angle of entry of the eustachian tube into the pharynx predisposes to tube closure by increasing pressure as descent continues. In babies and young children the angle of entry is less acute, and ear problems in flight are fewer. Upper respiratory tract infection, causing inflammation and oedema of the eustachian lining, increases the likelihood of otic barotrauma. In severe cases the tympanic membrane ruptures, with consequent relief of pain. Aircrew are made fully aware of this condition during training; if they are unable to clear their ears—for example during a cold—they are temporarily grounded. In doubtful cases a nonmoving tympanic membrane may be detected by direct vision. The toynbee manoeuvre is the best technique for evaluating eustachian function under physiological conditions at ground level: under direct vision, normal function is demonstrated by a slight inward movement of the tympanic membrane followed by a more marked outward movement. Because atmospheric pressure swings are greatest at low altitudes, passengers are often affected by tubal dysfunction. Education and instruction on the frenzel, toynbee, and valsalva manoeuvres help prevent much airborne misery, although some people have great difficulty in learning these procedures and some may be unable to do so even after much coaching and practice.

The treatment of otic barotrauma, particularly if blood or fluid is present in the middle ear cavity, should include analgesia, a nasal decongestant, and a broad spectrum antibiotic.

The cause of sinus barotrauma is the same as its otic counterpart. On ascent, expanding air vents easily from the sinuses through the ostia. On descent the ostia are readily occluded, especially if the subject has a cold. Characteristically a sudden very severe knife-like pain occurs in the affected sinus and epistaxis may result from submucosal haemorrhage. The condition is related to the rate of descent, and its prevention is part of the rationale behind the slow rates of descent of passenger aircraft. The possibility of a sinus problem cannot be predicted on the ground, but flying with a cold will increase the risk. Treatment should include a decongestant, analgesia, and a suitable antibiotic.

In summary, modern air travel is not without physiological hazards, and those described here are directly attributable to the

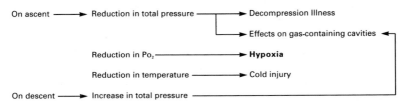

FIG 5.4—Physical changes in the atmosphere on ascent to and descent from altitude, and their clinical effects.

physical changes in the atmosphere inherent in ascent to high altitudes (fig 5.4).

1 *The Prayer Book* 1662; 18: 10.
2 Ernsting J. *Some effects of raised intrapulmonary pressure in man*. Maidenhead: Technivision Ltd, 1966.
3 Denison DM, Ledwith MA, Poulton EC. Complex reaction times at simulated cabin altitudes of 5000 feet and 8000 feet. *Aerospace Med* 1966; **37:** 1010–13.
4 Norris W. *The unsafe sky*. London: Arrow Books, 1981.
5 Underwood-Ground KE. Check your oxygen. *Aviat Space Environ Med* 1982; **53:** 24–6.
6 Ernsting J, Sharp GR (revised by Harding RM). Hypoxia and hyperventilation. In: Ernsting J, King PF, eds. *Aviation medicine*. 2nd edn. London: Butterworths, 1988: 48.
7 Harding RM. Molecular sieve oxygen concentrators in military aircraft. *Aeromed Training Digest* 1990; **4:** 47–54.
8 Hoffler GW, Turner HS, Wick RL, Billings CE. Behaviour of naive subjects during rapid decompression from 8000 to 30 000 feet. *Aerospace Med* 1974; **45:** 117–22.
9 von Beckh HJ. Forward facing versus rearward facing passenger seats during emergency descent of multi mach-high altitude transport aircraft. *Aerospace Med* 1969; **40:** 1215–18.
10 Perutz MF. Haemoglobin structure and respiratory transport. *Sci Am* 1978; **239:** 68–86.
11 Balke B, Wells JG, Clark RT. In-flight hyperventilation in aircraft pilots. *J Aviat Med* 1957; **28:** 241–8.
12 Lum LC. Hyperventilation and anxiety state. *J R Soc Med* 1981; **74:** 1–4.
13 Callahan M. Hypoxic hazards of traditional paper bag rebreathing in hyperventilating patients. *Ann Emerg Med* 1989; **18:** 622–8.
14 Ernsting J. Decompression sickness in aviation. In: Busby DE, ed. *Recent advances in aviation medicine*. Dordrecht: D Reidel Publishing Company, 1970: 177–87.
15 Fryer DI. *Subatmospheric decompression sickness in man*. Slough: Technivision Services, 1969.
16 Francis JR. The classification of decompression illness. In: Pilmanis AA, ed. *Proceedings of the 1990 hypobaric decompression sickness workshop*. AL-SR-1992-0005. Air Force Systems Command Armstrong Laboratory, Texas, 1992: 489–93.
17 Dully FE. Central nervous system involvement following type I aviator's bends complicated by complacency. *Aviat Space Environ Med* 1975; **46:** 1186–7.
18 Neubauer JC, Dixon JP, Herndon CM. Fatal pulmonary decompression sickness: a case report. *Aviat Space Environ Med* 1988; **59:** 1181–4.
19 Black WR, DeHart RL. Decompression sickness: an increasing risk for the private pilot. *Aviat Space Environ Med* 1992; **63:** 200–2.
20 Furry DE, Reeves E, Beckman E. Relationships of SCUBA diving to the development of aviator's decompression sickness. *Aerospace Med* 1967; **38:** 825–8.
21 Sheffield PJ. Flying after diving guidelines: a review. *Aviat Space Environ Med* 1990; **61:** 1130–8.
22 Ministry of Defence (Navy). *BR 2806 Diving Manual*. London, HMSO: 1972 (as amended to change 6) Articles 5121 and 5122.
23 Blumkin D. Flying and diving—a unique health concern. *Flight Safety Foundation's human factors and aviation medicine* 1991; **Sept/Oct:** 21–8.
24 Szmyd L, McCall CM. Aviation dentistry. In: Armstrong HG, ed. *Aerospace medicine*. London: Baillière, Tindall and Cox Ltd, 1961.
25 Harding RM. ENT problems and the air traveller. *Travel Med Int* 1992; **10:** 98–100.
26 King PF. The eustachian tube and its significance in flight. *J Laryngol Otol* 1979; **93:** 659–78.

6
Acceleration

Man regularly performs the greatest of all experiments in gravitational physiology at least once a day when he rises from his bed.[1]

Terrestrial life exposes us all to the acceleration of normal gravity for a lifetime. Flight and space exploration have, however, exposed humans to far greater accelerations which can be tolerated only for much shorter periods. The adverse physiological effects of these accelerations are fundamental problems in aviation medicine.

Acceleration is the rate of change of velocity with time and occurs when the speed or direction of motion of a body alters. The magnitude (nG) of an acceleration is conveniently expressed in multiples (n) of the acceleration due to gravity (g), which we sense as weight. Thus a military aircraft exposes its pilot to an acceleration of six times that of gravity when "pulling" 6 G, and the pilot's weight will consequently have increased sixfold. The pilot's physiological responses to this acceleration will be determined first by its magnitude and second by the duration and direction of its action. Duration of action may be classified as long or short, the time division between the two being set at 1 s. Although this separation appears to be quite arbitrary, in practice it is of great functional significance because excessive accelerations of short duration usually result in pathological changes, whereas those of long duration have physiological effects. The body responds to inertial force which, by Newton's third law of motion, is equal and opposite to the applied accelerative force. Thus the headwards acceleration of a pilot produces a footwards inertial force, and a car driver is flung forwards in a crash by a rearwards acting acceleration (equivalent to a forward deceleration). The body axis in which the inertial force acts is referred to as x (back–front), y (side–side), or z (head–foot) (fig 6.1).[2]

Long duration acceleration

In practice, linear accelerations of long duration produce no

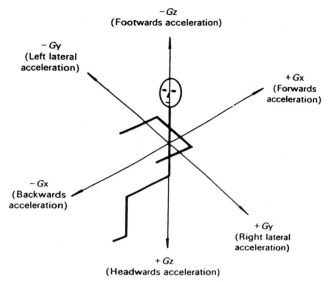

FIG 6.1—Inertial force vectors acting on the body: accelerative force acts in the opposite direction to inertial force.

important physiological effects because their magnitude and duration are both restricted by the speeds that can be attained on earth. In space flight, where velocity is less of a constraint, larger linear accelerations may produce significant physiological changes.

Radial accelerations of long duration are produced by a change in the direction of motion (as in manoeuvring an aircraft), and their duration may be limited only by fuel supply. In a conventional aircraft such accelerations act in the long axis of the body (Gz) and may be of sufficient magnitude to cause sustained distortion of structure and, more importantly, gross alterations in the flow and distribution of body fluids. If the head of the pilot is directed towards the centre of rotation then the inertial force is centrifugal (+ Gz), forcing the pilot down into the seat. Some military aircraft are now capable of sustaining accelerations of up to + 12 Gz without structural failure, but at such a high level of acceleration cerebral blood flow may be so reduced as to cause loss of consciousness, and the pilot is thus unable to control the aircraft. Advances in aeronautical engineering have challenged the acceleration physiologist to develop methods of protecting aircrew against the effects of + Gz acceleration. Such research requires the use of human-carrying centrifuges.

Physiology of + Gz acceleration

In an unprotected relaxed subject unconsciousness usually occurs between + 5 and + 6 Gz, the exact level depending on rate of onset of acceleration. If this is less than $2 \, G \, s^{-1}$ then the subject invariably experiences a sequence of visual symptoms before losing consciousness. At about + 3– + 4 Gz the visual fields become darker, and at 0·5–1 Gz later peripheral vision is lost. From this condition of "greyout" the fields contract further to a state of "blackout" and then vision is lost completely. Hearing and mental orientation are, however, adequate for intelligent conversation until consciousness is finally lost about 0·5 Gz after loss of vision. At higher rates of onset, progression to unconsciousness is too rapid for these characteristic visual symptoms to develop and may result in acceleration-induced loss of consciousness (G-LOC),[3] a phenomenon which has been cited as the cause of a number of fatal accidents and incidents in military fast jet aircraft.[4]

The cardinal determinant of these effects on vision and consciousness is cardiovascular. The arterial pressure of a fully reclined subject is essentially uniform throughout the body, but on standing—thereby changing the G vector from x to z—the subject's circulation is subjected to the action of hydrostatic forces. When a subject is upright blood in the vessels from the heart to the brain constitutes a column of fluid that at 1 Gz exerts a hydrostatic pressure of about 3·3 kPa (25 mmHg) (the pressure exerted by a column of fluid is equal to the product of its height, the density of the fluid, and the gravitational force). A mean arterial pressure of 13·3 kPa (100 mmHg) at the level of the heart would thus be decreased to 10·0 kPa (75 mmHg) at the level of the brain. Conversely, pressures below the level of the heart are increased by the hydrostatic pressure. Based on these figures the mean arterial pressure at brain level would be expected to be zero at + 4 Gz because the hydrostatic pressure opposing flow would be increased fourfold to 13·3 kPa (100 mmHg). Consciousness is, however, rarely lost below + 5 Gz, which suggests the anomaly of perfusion without pressure. In fact, flow is maintained because both the cerebrospinal fluid and the venous system are subject to the same hydrostatic laws as the arterial circulation. In animals exposed to + Gz acceleration cerebrospinal fluid and arterial pressures fall in unison[5] so that the pressure across the walls of the cerebral vessels may be expected to remain constant during the acceleration. This implies that the flow is determined solely by the difference in arteriovenous pressure. Because venous pressure also falls in parallel with arterial pressure a pressure gradient may be maintained, even with zero arterial pressure, provided that the jugular veins do not collapse when their internal pressure falls to subatmospheric levels. Even though pressures as low as -5.3 kPa (-40 mmHg) have been recorded from deep neck veins in humans exposed to $+4.5$ Gz,[6] the "jugular suction effect" cannot completely explain the preservation of consciousness. Undoubtedly, cerebral autoregulation is an important factor and, although this is difficult to investigate technically, there is evidence that cortical blood flow is maintained at the expense of less vital white matter.[7] A selective reduction in blood flow to the visual cortex is not, however, the basis of the visual symptoms, whose cause is peripheral.[8] The intraocular pressure of about 2.7 kPa (20 mmHg) will abolish retinal blood flow so as to cause "blackout" when arterial pressure falls below this value, although cerebral perfusion will continue. At the earlier "greyout" stage, the peripheral retina becomes hypoxic because of underperfusion due to reduced pressure in the retinal end arteries.

Because of raised hydrostatic pressures in the vessels below the level of the heart blood pools in the legs and abdomen, thereby reducing venous return and impairing cardiac output. The physiological changes produced by acceleration resemble those of haemorrhage, and both conditions cause similar reflex sympathetic responses—notably tachycardia and selective vasoconstriction. In humans the carotid sinus reflex is almost certainly responsible for the tachycardia but has little effect in inducing vasoconstriction.[9] Atrial pressure receptors, mesenteric baroreceptors, and local vessel response may all stimulate vasoconstriction secondary to haemorrhage in animals, but their role in humans has not been fully established.

Although hydrostatic pressures increase instantaneously with the onset of acceleration, reflex compensation takes at least 6 s to become effective. Thus it cannot prevent visual symptoms or unconsciousness developing except at very low rates of onset of acceleration, but it may improve visual symptoms already present. Sympathetic compensation is a basic accompaniment of orthostasis, so it is not surprising that anti-G trousers designed to benefit aircrew in the hypotensive environment of high $+Gz$ acceleration may be used to support patients with autonomic dysfunction. The pulmonary circulation is also affected by the increased hydrostatic pressure gradients of $+Gz$ acceleration. During such acceleration the lung apex, already poorly perfused at $+1$ Gz (normal gravity), is further compromised so that the alveolar dead space is increased. Below this point the rate at which blood flow per unit lung volume rises with distance down the lung increases with acceleration. Simultaneously, the weight of the lung rises in proportion to the force applied so that apical alveoli are stretched towards their maximum capacity and basal alveoli are compressed towards their minimum volume, thus encouraging airway closure. The overall effect of these changes is to intensify ventilation–perfusion inequalities and to produce large right-to-left shunts at the lung base, thereby reducing arterial oxygen saturation and aggravating cerebral hypoxia.[10] If the gas trapped at the lung base by airway closure is pure oxygen, as is supplied to military pilots at altitudes exceeding about 9144 m (30 000 ft), then basal collapse (atelectasis) may occur because of the attendant absorption of oxygen. This does not happen when air is breathed because of the presence in the closed off alveoli of inert, poorly absorbed nitrogen. The risk of oxygen atelectasis is greatly increased by inflation of anti-G trousers which, by raising the diaphragm, make the pilot breathe at a lower lung volume and therefore encourage the trapping of gas. Fortunately, rapid recovery takes place when the pressure in the airways is raised to a level exceeding critical opening pressure by a deep breath or cough.[11]

Protection against $+Gz$ acceleration

Tolerance to $+Gz$ acceleration, as measured by the levels at which visual symptoms develop in a "relaxed" subject riding on a centrifuge, may be increased by the pilot's voluntary action or by the passive use of purpose built equipment. Active straining will reduce cerebral hypotension by directly transmitting raised intrathoracic pressure to the arterial tree and, if combined with tensing of the limb muscles, will reduce the peripheral pooling of blood. Indeed, military pilots titrate the effectiveness of these anti-G straining manoeuvres against the visual changes experienced as high $+Gz$ acceleration builds up. An undesirable consequence of a sustained increase in intrathoracic pressure (as occurs with a valsalva manoeuvre) is impairment of venous return which, by depressing cardiac output, results in hypotension. Forced expiration against a *partially* closed glottis (the M-1 procedure) is therefore the voluntary action of choice because the necessary inspiratory phase permits venous return to recover. It is repeated every 3–4 s and may raise the visual threshold by up to $+2$ Gz but it produces fatigue and interferes with communication, disadvantages which do not occur with passive protection.[12]

The simplest method of passive protection is to reduce the vertical distance between the pilot's eye and heart by reclining the seat away from the vertical; an angle of 55° gives a benefit of about 1 G,[13] and a few combat aircraft—such as the General Dynamics F16—are fitted with modestly reclined seats. Nevertheless, the perennial method of passive protection is anti-G trousers, which raise tolerance by up to $+1.5$ Gz. Anti-G trousers are made of inextensible fabric containing interconnecting air bladders over the abdomen and legs. An acceleration-sensitive valve inflates the bladders to a pressure of 8–7 kPa (65 mmHg) per G, thereby applying counter pressure to the lower body, which reduces peripheral pooling of blood. This action alone cannot explain the sudden improvement in tolerance seen with inflation because sequestration of blood takes some seconds to develop. Inflation does, however, produce an immediate increase in peripheral resistance by the mechanical constriction of arterioles[14] and the raised intra-abdominal pressure lifts the heart upwards, thus reducing the vertical distance between eye and heart.[15]

The next generation of high performance military aircraft will have such agility that the now accepted limits of human tolerance to increased accelerations will be easily exceeded. This has led to intensive research into additional methods of improving tolerance. Thus, it has been established that extending the area of the lower body covered by the bladder of anti-G trousers will improve relaxed tolerance by an average of $+2.5$ Gz.[16] When this is combined with the automatic and progressive elevation of intra-thoracic pressure during excursions above $+4$ Gz—positive pressure breathing for G protection—pilot performance (again, as measured by relaxed tolerance) can be relatively easily maintained at sustained levels of acceleration as high as $+8–8.5$ Gz.[16] With minimal muscle tensing, tolerance can be extended to $+9$ Gz and when this technique is supplemented by a full anti-G straining manoeuvre performance can be maintained at levels in excess of $+10$ Gz for short periods. Positive pressure breathing used in this way at moderate levels of acceleration provides a passive replacement for anti-G straining manoeuvres, and so is much less fatiguing. The introduction of extended coverage anti-G trousers in combination with positive pressure breathing offers the best possibility so far of reducing the incidence of acceleration-induced loss of consciousness.[17]

Physiology of − Gz acceleration

Certain aerobatic manoeuvres—for example outside loops—produce − Gz acceleration, where the pilot's head is directed away from the centre of rotation. It is subjectively unpleasant, and the only practical method of protection is to avoid those manoeuvres which produce it.

Predictably, the cardiovascular effects are the opposite of those of + Gz acceleration. Vascular pressures increase above the heart and stimulate a bradycardia via the carotid sinus reflex.[18] In extreme cases asystole can lead to unconsciousness, a "physiologically normal" pressure being maintained despite cessation of circulation. Pooling of blood in the facial and neck tissues produces an unpleasant engorged feeling, but cerebral haemorrhage does not occur because of the protective effect of the parallel increase in cerebrospinal fluid pressure. Occasionally, pilots describe a red misting of vision ("redout") after − Gz exposure; this is not due to retinal haemorrhage (which would produce blindness) but is probably secondary to staining of tears with blood from conjunctival haemorrhage.[19]

Short duration acceleration

Abrupt decelerations commonly occur in accidents, whereas abrupt accelerations are more usual in military procedures—for example during ejection from aircraft. Both produce effects that depend on the mechanical strength of body tissues. These effects have been investigated experimentally by the use of test rigs which produce controlled impacts, but because experiments on human volunteers must be stopped before irreversible injury occurs, much information depends on the investigation of accidents or on studies of animals and anthropometric dummies. Accurate measurement of acceleration is complicated and, ideally, triaxial linear and angular accelerometers should be used. In addition, the different densities and dynamic characteristics of the tissues imply that measured accelerations may differ greatly between various parts of the body. These factors, together with a wide range of individual variation and the importance of other variables such as body restraint, mean that tolerance limits should be interpreted with care.

Assessing tolerance to impact

The criteria used to define tolerance depend on the circumstances of the impact: at one extreme, survival after an aircraft crash—even with serious injury—would be acceptable, while at the other—for example in a decision on the maximum force that an escalator may impart to a passenger's foot—any injury would be unacceptable. Tolerance will also be affected if the impact is directed towards a particular area of the body: a kick in the buttock is less damaging than an equivalent blow to the nape of the neck. In aviation medical research on impact, however, the prime concern is with the response of the whole body.

The injury potential of an impact is determined particularly by the induced velocity change so that as the duration of the acceleration is decreased higher peak acceleration levels may be tolerated.[20] This explains why, in a forward facing impact ($-Gx$) with adequate restraint of the upper half of the body, tolerance is reduced from 45 G for a duration of 0·1 s to 25 G for a duration of 0·2 s.[21] Short duration accelerations are also complicated by the rate of onset of acceleration (jolt), because a higher jolt may lead to a dynamic overshoot with resultant increases in local forces. For example, Stapp[22] found that a peak acceleration of about $-38·6$ Gx for 0·28 s produced no signs of shock when the jolt was 314 G s^{-1}, but at a peak of $-38·5$ Gx for 0·16 s severe shock was produced at a jolt of 1315 G s^{-1}. In a rearward facing impact ($+Gx$) one of Stapp's group managed to survive a voluntary insult of $+40$ Gx for 0·04 s at a jolt of 2139 G s^{-1}. Body orientation therefore appears to have an appreciable influence on tolerance, because such an impact would not have been endured in a forward facing seat.

The importance of body orientation and restraint on human tolerance to horizontal impacts is outlined in fig 6.2. When an upright subject is unrestrained, tolerance—as defined by forward motion—is very low and depends on the subject's ability to maintain posture by muscular effort. Tolerance is increased in this orientation if a suitable immovable object can be gripped, but it remains well below that in subjects supported by a seat. By bracing

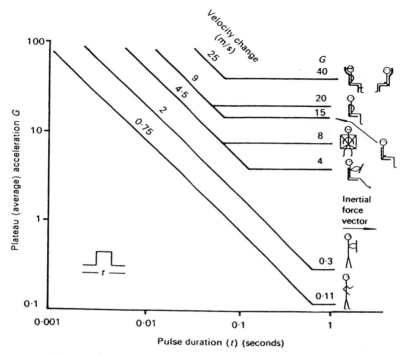

FIG 6.2—Human tolerance to horizontal impact in attitudes and restraints indicated by the matchstick figures. The logarithm of acceleration has been plotted against the logarithm of the duration of the acceleration pulse, which has been assumed to be rectangular. (Although most impact acceleration pulses are shaped like an inverted V or U, a rectangular form is an acceptable compromise.) Below a certain pulse duration tolerance is determined by velocity change but beyond this point acceleration levels (G, right of graph) become critical. (Reproduced by permission of group captain D Glaister.)

against the steering wheel an unrestrained driver may prevent forward motion up to a level of − 4 Gx. Tolerance may be further improved only by applying passive restraint over as large an area as possible or to a portion of the body well adapted to tolerating high local pressure such as bone.

Preventing injury

The simplest form of restraint, as worn by airline passengers, is a lap strap, which when correctly positioned should lie over the anterior superior iliac spines. Although tolerance is increased the

81

subject's body may jack-knife over the belt, striking structures in front: indeed, deaths have occurred at otherwise survivable levels of impact simply because the head has struck sharp forward structures. In addition, submarining (rotation of the pelvis under the strap) may occur and increase the risk of injury to the abdominal organs and lumbar spine because of the high local loads. Jack-knifing may be eliminated by adding an upper torso restraint to the lap strap, but submarining may be effectively overcome only by adding a so called "negative strap" that runs between the legs to connect the centre of the strap to the seat.

Increasing the area over which the decelerative force is applied improves tolerance by reducing the load per unit area. This may be achieved by increasing restraint or, more effectively, by using a rearward facing seat. Such a seat, with a lap restraint to prevent the subject from rebounding out of it, may increase tolerance to levels seen only in forward facing impacts ($-Gx$) when the head, arms, and legs are restrained as well as the upper half of the body.[20,23] Because of the higher loading on the seat back, rearward-facing seats and their floor attachments need to be strengthened.

For the past 45 years both the Royal Air Force and the United States Air Force have fitted only rearward facing seats in their transport aircraft, which has demonstrably improved survival in accidents.[24,25] This idea has still not been adopted by commercial airlines because of increased cost and weight, and possible consumer rejection. Recently, however, stronger seats have been developed without imposing weight penalties, and it is by no means certain that passengers would object to rearward facing seats.[25]

Lateral accelerations (Gy) are usually less well tolerated than those in the x axis because neck injury may occur at quite low acceleration loads. However, if the head is fully restrained tolerance levels are similar in both axes.[20,26]

Aviation medical interest in short duration vertical accelerations was stimulated by the need for rapid escape from military aircraft which is achieved by expelling the crew member on the seat by explosive charges. The major factor limiting the acceleration profile imposed by the ejection seat is overloading of the spine with resultant compression fracture, most commonly of T12 and L1 vertebrae,[27] where the cross-sectional area is smallest. Various degrees of spinal damage occur in up to half of all ejectees, but these are acceptable when the alternative is to remain within a doomed aircraft.[28] Spinal injury may be reduced by engineering factors such as a reduction in jolt; and this can be achieved by using multiple small explosive charges rather than a few large ones and rocket motors to extend the time over which the force is applied.

In the final analysis the problem of improving tolerance to short duration accelerations has to be solved by the engineer with the knowledge of human limits and injury mechanisms gained by acceleration physiologists and pathologists.

1 Howard P. Gravity and the circulation. *Proc R Soc Lond (Biol)* 1977; **199:** 485–91.
2 Gell CF. Table of equivalents for acceleration terminology. *Aerospace Med* 1961; **32:** 1109–11.
3 Burton RR. G-induced loss of consciousness: definition, history, current status. *Aviat Space Environ Med* 1988; **59:** 2–5.
4 Lyons TJ, Harding RM, Freeman J, Oakley C. G-induced loss of consciousness accidents: USAF experience 1982–1990. *Aviat Space Environ Med* 1992; **63:** 60–6.
5 Rushmer RF, Beckman EL, Lee D. Protection of the cerebral circulation by the cerebrospinal fluid under the influence of radial acceleration. *Am J Physiol* 1947; **151:** 355–65.
6 Henry JP, Gauer OH, Kety SS, Kramer K. Factors maintaining cerebral circulation during gravitational stress. *J Clin Invest* 1951; **30:** 292–300.
7 Howard P, Glaister DH. The effects of positive acceleration upon cerebral blood flow. *J Physiol* 1964; **171:** 39P.
8 Duane TD. Observations on the fundus oculi during black-out. *Arch Ophthalmol* 1954; **51:** 343–55.
9 Roddie IC, Shepherd JT. Some effects of carotid artery compression in man with special reference to changes in vascular resistance in the limbs. *J Physiol* 1957; **139:** 377–84.
10 Glaister DH. The effects of gravity and acceleration on the lung. *Advisory Group for Aerospace Research and Development (AGARDograph No 133)*. Slough: Technician Services, 1970.
11 Glaister DH. Lung collapse in aviation medicine. *Br J Hosp Med* 1969; **2:** 635–42.
12 Burton RR, Leverett SD, Michaelson ED. Man at high sustained +Gz acceleration: a review. *Aerospace Med* 1974; **45:** 1115–36.
13 Burns JW. Re-evaluation of a tilt-back seat as a means of increasing acceleration tolerance. *Aviat Space Environ Med* 1975; **46:** 55–63.
14 Wood EH, Lambert EH. Some factors which influence the protection afforded by pneumatic anti-G suits. *J Aviat Med* 1952; **23:** 218–28.
15 Rushmer RF. A roentgenographic study of the effect of a pneumatic anti-blackout suit on the hydrostatic columns in man exposed to positive radial acceleration. *Am J Physiol* 1947; **151:** 459–68.
16 Green NDC. The physiological limitations of man in the high G environment. In: *Combat automation for airborne weapons systems: man–machine interface trends and technologies.* Neuilly-sur-Seine, France: NATO Advisory Group for Aerospace Research and Development, 1993; AGARD Conference Proceedings No 250: 17.1–17.8.
17 Harding RM, Bomar JB. Positive pressure breathing for acceleration protection and its role in the prevention of inflight G-induced loss of consciousness. *Aviat Space Environ Med* 1990; **61:** 845–9.
18 Gauer OH, Henry JP. Negative (−Gz) acceleration in relation to arterial oxygen saturation, subendocardial haemorrhage and venous pressure in the forehead. *Aerospace Med* 1964; **34:** 533–45.
19 Howard P. Acceleration. In: Edholm OG, Weiner JS, eds. *The principles and practice of human physiology.* London: Academic Press, 1981: 203–4.
20 Glaister DH. Human tolerance to impact acceleration. *Injury* 1978; **9:** 191–8.
21 Snyder RG. Impact. In: Parker JF, West VR, eds. *Bioastronautics data book*, 2nd edn. Houston, Texas: National Aeronautics and Space Administration, 1973: 229 (SP-3006).
22 Stapp JP. Voluntary human tolerance limits. In: Gurdjian ES, Lange WA, Patrick LM, Thomas LM, eds. *Impact injury and crash protection.* Springfield, IL: Charles C Thomas, 1970: 319, 329.

23 Fryer DI. Passenger survival in aircraft crashes. *Aeronautics* 1959; **40**: 31–7.
24 Campbell HE. The case for rear facing seats in commercial aircraft. *Clin Med* 1960; **67**: 2529–37.
25 Snyder RG. Advanced techniques in crash impact protection and emergency egress from air transport aircaft. *Advisory Group for Aerospace Research and Development (AGARDograph No 221)*. London: Technical Editing and Reproduction Ltd, 1976: 66–9.
26 Weis EB, Clarke NP, Brinkley JW. Human response to several impact acceleration orientations and patterns. *Aerospace Med* 1963; **34**: 1122–9.
27 Auffret R, Delahaye RP. Spinal injury after ejection. *Advisory Group for Aerospace Research and Development Advisory Report No 72*. London: Technical Editing and Reproduction Ltd, 1975.
28 Anton DJ. Aircrew safety and survivability (limited to combat aircraft): survival after ejection 1968–1979. *Advisory Group for Aerospace Research and Development Conference Proceedings No 286*. London: Technical Editing and Reproduction Ltd, 1980: A8.1–A8.4.

7
Function of the special senses in flight

Who needs instruments said he, with perfect eyesight like me?
My approach seems just right, he thought one black night,
And calmly flew into the sea.

Anon

The special senses are vital to safe flying; the visual, vestibular, and auditory modalities are particularly important, but even touch and smell have a role to play. This chapter is concerned with the way in which the senses operate in, and may be adversely affected by, the abnormal environment of flight.

Vision

Perfect eyesight is indispensable to pilots but, even with excellent vision, flight imposes certain peculiarly visual limitations and problems. In high speed flight (greater than 450 knots), particularly at very low level (altitudes below 153 m (500 ft)), the principal problem is extension of the total reaction time. For a human–machine complex this is conventionally divided into phases of perception (pickup, lockon, recognition), evaluation, decision, action, and response. Under perfect conditions it lasts 5–7 s: a timespan that represents a distance travelled of nearly 2 miles (~3 km) for two aircraft flying on a collision course at a combined speed of about 1800 kph (1120 mph). The greatest distance at which any target might be expected to be seen—and only then as a point source without discernible detail—is about 11 km (6·8 miles),[1] so anything which extends the total reaction time will jeopardise the aircraft and its occupants. Although many factors—including workload and fatigue—may prolong this period, the initial triggering of the "visual perception cascade" of pickup, lockon and recognition is especially important.[2]

85

This phase occupies about 1 s under ideal circumstances, but visual factors which delay the cascade will prolong the total reaction time accordingly: these include poor atmospheric conditions (haze, fog, cloud), night flying, and the size and contrast of the target (small, camouflaged aircraft will be seen later than large, well lit or brightly coloured machines). The dynamic visual field also has an effect: targets approaching head on stimulate the retina less than those tracking tangentially across the visual field and so delay pickup.

High altitude flight—that is, at altitudes above 12 192 m (40 000 ft)—produces other visual problems, including solar glare.[3] There is a slight increase in the intensity of light as altitude increases to 30 480 m (100 000 ft), and its distribution is so modified at altitude that most appears to come from below, where scattering of light by air molecules, moisture, and dust particles is greater and where clouds may create a bright visual floor. Therefore at altitude the sky above appears darker, less light falls on the cockpit interior—particularly on the instrument panels—and the degree of contrast is increased so that retinal adaptation time is prolonged when the pilot looks from inside the cockpit to outside or vice versa. Colour discrimination is also affected by glare, which may be reduced by wearing sunglasses or by attaching a tinted visor to the helmets of military aircrew. High intensity cockpit instrument lighting, which reduces excessive contrast, has been fitted in some aircraft.

Visual function may be further impaired at altitude by the development of empty visual field myopia. In this condition there is no external detail on which the eye can focus—for example in a cloudless sky at high altitude, in total darkness, or in a uniformly overcast sky—and the eye is unable to focus at infinity and instead remains in a steady state of activity focused 1–2 m (3–6 ft) away. In this case the size of a target that is visible when the ability to focus at infinity is intact has to be doubled to be detected, thus increasing the duration of the visual cascade.[4] Pilots are taught to minimise the risks associated with empty visual fields by periodically and deliberately focusing on an object known to be effectively at infinity, such as the wing tip.

At night, empty visual field myopia may be further complicated by the need to use off-centre scanning techniques to ensure that dimly lit external targets are not missed by foveal scanning. Such off-centre vision is effective only if the eye is fully adapted to the dark and about 30 min is needed for the rods to achieve maximum scotopic sensitivity.[5] Historically, adaptation to the dark began on the ground with the use of red goggles and was maintained in the air by red cockpit lighting. This degree of adaptation is no longer considered necessary because night flight requires photopic function both for monitoring instruments and for accomplishing most external visual tasks. Red lighting is now felt to be inappropriate, because it also impairs colour discrimination and reduces accommodative ability and speed. Dim white general lighting has none of these disadvantages and is preferred.[6]

Ocular hazards of a physical kind, such as windblast on ejection and birdstrikes, are important in military aviation. For these reasons military aircrew are usually provided with a helmet-mounted clear polycarbonate visor in addition to, but operated independently of, the tinted visor, which is lowered during low altitude flight and if possible before ejection. The aircrew helmet is also increasingly used as a mounting platform for vision enhancing devices, such as target designators and night vision goggles. With regard to the latter, it has long been recognised that unassisted night vision is inadequate for military purposes, and so image intensifier tubes (which amplify reflected residual light in the longer visible and near infrared part of the spectrum) have been developed with increasing sophistication and performance. Not surprisingly, however, night vision goggles produce visual problems of their own including loss of peripheral vision, reduction in contrast, absence of colour discrimination, and impairment of depth perception and judgement of distance. Also, even with modern devices, visual acuity is degraded from the normal aircrew standard of 6/6 to 6/9–6/12.

Finally, visual mechanisms are of paramount relevance to orientation and disorientation.

Spatial orientation and disorientation

The organs of spatial orientation are the means by which position, attitude, and movement are determined in relation to fixed references. On the ground, the references are gravity and the horizon, and it is in this 1 G environment that the perception of correct orientation develops, based on information from the eyes, inner ear, and proprioceptors. Once the pilot is airborne and subject to abnormal accelerative forces, however, the information supplied by these sensory modalities—particularly the vestibular apparatus and proprioceptors—may be interpreted incorrectly with potentially dangerous consequences. Correct spatial orientation is replaced by spatial *dis*orientation in which the pilot's perception of his or her own position (and often that of the aircraft) is false.[7] All aircrew experience disorientation at some stage during their careers, but it is only when control of the aircraft is based on false perceptions that accidents occur.

Disorientation was implicated in about 12% of all British airline accidents during the period 1978–1988,[8] and a similar figure has been derived for fixed wing aircraft accidents in the Royal Air Force over the period 1973–1991. In the United States Air Force, 14% of such accidents were attributed to spatial disorientation during 1989–1991.[9] However, the extent of the problem is hidden by the bland use of percentages: in the United States Air Force over the 10 year period 1980–1989, "conventional" spatial disorientation was cited as the major cause in 81 of 633 accidents (13%), and was responsible for 115 of the 795 resulting fatalities, at a material cost of $539 million. When combined with citations of a closely related phenomenon, termed loss of situational awareness, in which channelised attention, distraction, or task saturation are manifest, the statistics reveal that spatial disorientation and loss of situational awareness were responsible for 270 (43%) of the 633 accidents and 437 deaths for a material cost of over $2 billion! In view of these horrifying figures, it is perhaps surprising that research into spatial disorientation/loss of situational awareness has not attracted more attention, finance and effort; particularly when compared to the problem of acceleration-induced loss of consciousness (see chapter 6) which has been the subject of intense and very expensive research activity around the world, yet which caused just 18 accidents and 14 deaths (albeit 14 too many) in the United States Air Force during the period 1982–1990.[10]

Spatial disorientation is also the cause of many rotary wing accidents (see also chapter 11) being cited as the cause, for example, of up to 21% and 14% in the British Army and the United States Army respectively.[11,12] The world of general aviation is also affected: one study cited spatial disorientation as a cause (or contributory cause) of 2·5% of all accidents in this class and 16% of fatal accidents during the period 1968–1975,[13] but the actual figure is probably much higher.

Mechanism of orientation

If visual function is normal and external cues unambiguous, vision provides reliable sensory information from which orientation may be perceived correctly. Similarly, the semicircular canals provide reliable information about angular acceleration of the head and may be regarded as angular accelerometers working as three matched pairs (fig 7.1). Sustained change in the angular velocity of the head greater than about $3°\,s^{-1}$ is detected by the canals in the plane of movement and its magnitude and direction are signalled to the brain. Movement will be detected by the canals only for as long as there is a suprathreshold acceleration or deceleration and once constant velocity is reached the signal will decay even though movement is continuing.[7] The otolith organs, which lie within the utricles and saccules and are also bilateral, are linear accelerometers: the utricles lie in the horizontal plane, the saccules in the vertical (fig 7.1). The otoliths register accelerations greater than $0·1\,m\,s^{-2}$, but again the signals decay when constant velocity is reached. Cerebral integration and interpretation of vestibular signals is achieved in conjunction with visual signals and is reinforced by proprioceptive information to produce a complete and accurate assessment of body orientation.

The principal function of the vestibular apparatus is, however, the maintenance of body equilibrium by reflex motor control of muscle groups. The most important group in relation to orientation is the ocular musculature. Vestibular stabilisation of this

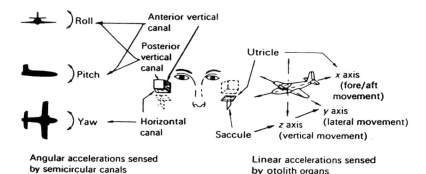

FIG 7.1—Relation of the components of the vestibular apparatus to their axes of response and to the planes of aircraft movement.

muscle group is responsible for the maintenance of a static retinal image whenever the head is moved. Thus every response of the semicircular canals, however small, is matched by compensatory eye movements that are equal in magnitude but opposite in direction to the movement of the head. Such vestibulo-ocular reflexes are also present in response to inputs from the otoliths but are less precise.

Once a person is exposed by flight to patterns of angular and linear motion beyond the dynamic range of sense organs adapted for life on the ground, visual, vestibular, and proprioceptive signals—which are further complicated by the vestibulo-ocular reflexes and by central mechanisms—may be totally erroneous and lead to false perceptions. These illusions may be classified by their system of origin but considerable overlap exists between them.

Illusions of visual origin

Pilots are taught to fly in accordance with regulations for visual flight, used when meteorological conditions exceed certain laid down minima, or for instrument flight, used at all other times.[14] When flying under visual flight rules, any impairment of vision may very quickly lead to catastrophic disorientation because it will require immediate transition to instrument rules. During the time taken to recognise the need for transition and to accomplish it the risk of disorientation is greatly increased. Thus absent or inadequate visual cues—as when flying in cloud, fog, rain, dust, at night, or over featureless landscapes such as sand, grass, or water—are particularly hazardous. The situation is dangerously compounded if there is also any failure of, or lag time in, the instrument displays, because the pilot relies on these when the external visual field is absent or impaired. Visual problems are accentuated even further by vibration, turbulence, or glare. Occasionally, despite an apparently normal external visual scene, visual cues may be falsely interpreted, usually as a result of errors of expectancy. For example, a sloping cloudbank may be assumed to be horizontal because most cloud tops are horizontal (fig 7.2).

Both visual impairment and errors of expectancy are particularly relevant during approach and landing, a phase of flight in which eight of the 15 British airline accidents in 1990 occurred.[15] Height and distance have to be accurately judged in the final stages of landings by means of several monocular visual cues including the shape of the runway and its changing perspective, motion parallax,

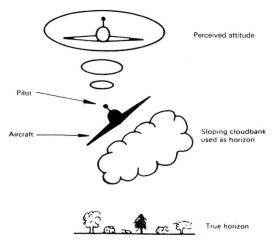

Perceived attitude

Pilot

Aircraft

Sloping cloudbank
used as horizon

True horizon

FIG 7.2—Error of expectancy: the sloping cloud bank is assumed to be horizontal.
(After Benson and Burchard.[7])

and retinal image size and movement. Any factor that interferes
with or modifies these cues may lead to mistakes. Landing in fog,
haze, rain, or at night may cause overestimation of height and
distance; landing in clear, bright conditions may cause under-
estimation. The attempt by the pilot to attain the expected
angle of approach of 2·5–3° under such circumstances may lead
to landing short of the runway if height and distance are over-
estimated and to landing long if they are underestimated. There
is little time in this phase of flight to correct mistakes.

A further purely visual illusion is the apparent movement of a
single static point source of light at night—the autokinetic illusion.
The absence of other detail in the visual field, combined with small
but normal involuntary eye and neck movements, leads to the
impression of movement of the light across the field of vision,
usually randomly but occasionally in a deliberate manner. The
pilot may take potentially dangerous avoiding action on the as-
sumption that the light is another aircraft.

Illusions of vestibular origin

As with visual information, that reaching the vestibular apparatus may be inadequate or erroneous. Movements in flight may be
so slight as to be subthreshold. (The thresholds quoted above for

91

angular and linear accelerations are laboratory findings but in flight they may be much higher because the pilot's attention is devoted to other aspects of flying.) Subthreshold phenomena are probably responsible for the most frequent form of disorientation: the so called "leans".[16] In this condition (fig 7.3) the aircraft and its pilot adopt an abnormal attitude—for example in roll—at a sub-subthreshold rate. A pilot may recognise the situation by referring to instruments and will then correct the attitude, but at a supra-threshold rate. This movement, the first to be sensed by the semicircular canals, is interpreted by the brain as a movement in the opposite direction to the original, unsensed, change of attitude: the pilot knows from the instruments that the flight path is now straight and level but nevertheless feels that the aircraft is leaning to one side.

Erroneous information is also common. For example, the semicircular canals may provide false information on recovery from a prolonged spin. During the spin the canals correctly indicate an angular acceleration, but once constant velocity is reached the signal decays only to recur and indicate rotation in the opposite direction when the spin is recovered. The pilot feels that he has entered a spin in the opposite direction and may, because of the somatogyral illusion, re-enter the original spin in an attempt to counter the apparent new one. The vestibulo-ocular reflex then stimulates a postrotational nystagmus so that vision is impaired in parallel with the erroneous vestibular sensations. This visual component is called the oculogyral illusion.[17] Fortunately, any sensory conflict is usually resolved quickly, but in extreme and rare cases the cycle may repeat itself until the pilot, who is usually inexperienced, crashes at the end of what has become a "graveyard" spin.[18]

The semicircular canals may also produce false sensations of

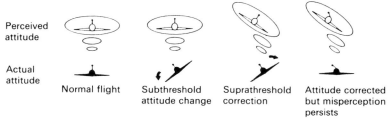

FIG 7.3—One mechanism by which the "leans" may be produced. (After Benson and Burchard.[7])

movement when the head is rotated while the aircraft is turning. This phenomenon, the coriolis effect, results from the introduction of a previously unstimulated pair of canals into the plane of movement. As a simple example, with the aircraft turning solely in yaw—a motion normally signalled by the horizontal canals—the head is rotated to the left and down to monitor an instrument. This manoeuvre brings the vertical canals into, and the horizontal canals out of, the plane of movement: there is acceleration of the former and deceleration of the latter and the complex signals from the whole apparatus create a bizarre vertigo in which the dominant illusory sensation is one of rotation in pitch.

Similar false sensations of angular movement may be precipitated by pressure changes transmitted from the middle ear cavity to the labyrinth via the round window. Such pressure changes are usually symmetrical, but if they should be unequal because of eustachian dysfunction then pressure or alternobaric vertigo may result.[19] This uncommon condition is a further reason for the temporary grounding of aircrew with upper respiratory tract infections.

Linear accelerations are transduced by the otolith organs and proprioceptors and then interpreted by the brain. The brain does not, however, distinguish between imposed linear acceleration and acceleration due to gravity and regards their resultant perception as the true vertical. This perceptual limitation leads to somatogravic or pitch illusions (fig 7.4).[7] Sustained forward acceleration ($+Gx$), as on take off, creates an inertial force which pushes the pilot back into the seat. When combined with gravity ($+1\ Gz$) the resultant force is inclined backwards but the pilot's brain interprets this as the true vertical and the pilot feels that the aircraft is in a nose up attitude. The vestibulo-ocular reflex produces an oculogravic effect, which confirms the sensation of pitch by generating a visual field that is also pitching. The pilot's instinctive response is to correct the error by lowering the nose of the aircraft, an action that could be disastrous. The opposite situation occurs during sustained decelerations—for example, when air brakes are applied. Thus at vital stages of flight the pitch illusions may have a catastrophic effect.

Illusions of cerebral origin

Correct sensory information may be misinterpreted by the brain—for example, causing errors of expectancy—but coning of

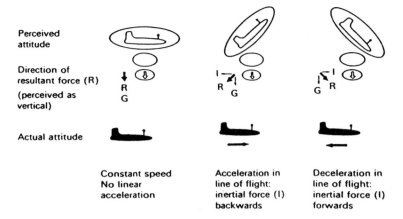

Perceived attitude

Direction of resultant force (R) (perceived as vertical)

Actual attitude

| Constant speed No linear acceleration | Acceleration in line of flight: inertial force (I) backwards | Deceleration in line of flight: inertial force (I) forwards |

FIG 7.4—Mechanisms by which pitch or somatogravic illusions may be produced (G, acceleration due to gravity). (After Benson and Burchard.[7])

attention (fascination), high or low arousal states, and other environmental stresses such as hypoxia and hyperthermia also affect the central nervous system. The breakoff phenomenon is, however, a purely central cause of disorientation in which the victim is subject to bizarre sensations of dissociation. This usually occurs when the sensorium is relatively unoccupied and unstimulated, as in straight and level flight at high altitude. Aircrew must be made aware of the possibility of such dissociative sensations under these circumstances lest they believe them to have a psychiatric basis.[20]

Spatial disorientation must be regarded as an extension of normal physiology, which implies that it cannot be entirely prevented. The risks may be minimised if the predisposing factors are known. Operational aircrew must be taught to recognise those environments (night, fog, cloud), phases (landing, take off, high altitude), and manoeuvres (spins, head movements) which may lead to disorientation, and to be particularly alert at these times. They must also learn to reject bodily sensations as unreliable. Within the aircraft itself clear, adequate, unambiguous, and reliable instrumentation should be located so as to avoid unnecessary head movement.

Aircrew must be fit to fly and have no acute or chronic sensory disorder. The deleterious effects of hypoxia, heat, exercise, fatigue, cigarettes, drugs, and alcohol must be emphasised during training. Training itself and experience are invaluable assets, although even highly experienced aircrew are not immune from disorientation.[21]

Motion sickness

The principal clinical features of motion sickness are familiar to most people, and consist of epigastric discomfort followed by increasing nausea, pallor, and sweating. The condition may then rapidly worsen (the "avalanche phenomenon"), with increased salivation, feelings of warmth, and emesis. Secondary, less common features may include hyperventilation, frontal headache, flatulence, depression, and drowsiness.

Why should motion produce such a reaction, because this syndrome (usually, but not necessarily, culminating in emesis) constitutes a poison-response mechanism which is normally activated within the central nervous system as a protective reaction to the ingestion of toxic substances? Many theories have been advanced to explain the phenomenon, of which two have particular appeal.

The first, Reason's neural mismatch (conflict) theory, provides a pragmatic and mechanistically useful model to explain why certain motion stimuli produce motion sickness but others do not.[22] It also accounts for the occurrence of sickness when certain expected motion cues are absent—for example inflight simulators—and suggests that, when motion sickness develops, the sensory information provided by the visual, vestibular, and proprioceptive apparatus is at variance with that expected on the basis of experience. The mismatch not only leads to sickness but also initiates changes within the central nervous system that are responsible for the development of protective adaptation. The conflict theory does not, however, explain why motion sickness takes the form that it does or why it should occur at all.

To explain this aspect, Treisman has extended the conflict theory by postulating that the brainstem mechanisms responsible for orientation and motion are also responsible for the detection of, and response to, poisoning.[23] Thus motion sickness occurs when sensory inputs to the brainstem are so confusing as to mimic the ingestion of poison. There is convincing evidence that this is so: surgical removal of the vestibular apparatus in experimental animals renders them not only immune to motion sickness but also unresponsive to certain poisons.[24]

Thus, motion *sickness* is really a misnomer because it is a normal manifestation of sensory function in response to real or apparent (that is, absent), but unfamiliar, motion stimuli. It is also the activation, by motion, of a primitive response to poison.[25] Its incidence varies with the motion environment: among those in liferafts in heavy sea states almost 99% are affected, but in civil aircraft the incidence is usually well below 1% and rises to only about 8% in severe turbulence. It also occurs in significant numbers in environments where expected motion cues are absent, for example in simulators (10–60%)[26] or large screen (Imax) cinemas.

In military aviation the problem of motion sickness is very real and has been responsible for failure during flying training of many hopeful aircrew: in 1942, for example, 11% of United States Navy trainees developed air sickness, and 52% of those failed their training course.[27] In the United Kingdom 20 years ago, up to 40% of trainees were afflicted: 15% to a degree which compromised performance.[28] More recently, a large longitudinal study, again in the United States Navy but this time of non-pilot aircrew in training, revealed that about 13·5% were affected to a degree that degraded flying performance: the percentage was greatest during basic training (19%) and fell thereafter to just under 12% during advanced training and to 7·6% during flight readiness sorties.[29] It is a feature of increased flying experience (adaptation) that motion sickness becomes less of a problem with time.[30]

Motion sickness in aircrew is best prevented by protective adaptation through repeated exposure to provocative motion environments; also by good postural stability within the aircraft, good control dynamics, sound ergonomic design, and avoiding unpleasant environmental conditions such as heat and odours. Those aircrew affected by persistent airsickness, usually during basic training or after reassignment to a different aircraft type, may be salvaged by a programme of desensitisation and rehabilitation. Such programmes may involve a phase of adaptation to ground-based nauseogenic stimuli (with or without reinforcement by biofeedback and relaxation techniques) followed by an airborne phase during which increasingly provocative flight profiles are flown.[31] They are undoubtedly cost effective and may return to active flying duties 80–90% of those trainee aircrew who would otherwise have been lost.[32]

In passengers, pharmacological prophylaxis is a more realistic approach. None of the currently available drugs—including hyoscine (scopolamine), cyclizine, dimenhydrinate, and promethazine—is, however, fully effective and, as central cholinergic blockers, all have central and/or autonomic side effects. This also includes cinnarizine, which it was originally believed rarely caused drowsiness when used for seasickness.[33] Drowsiness does occur, however, but usually after about 5 hours: indeed, if taken well before (about 4 hours) exposure to motion cinnarizine can be as effective as hyoscine. If it is taken 2 hours before exposure there may be little or no benefit.[34] Comparative drug studies have generally concluded that hyoscine is the most effective single preparation for both the prophylaxis and the treatment of motion sickness.[35] The effectiveness of transdermal hyoscine is similar to that of the oral preparation but has the additional advantages of ease of use and long duration of action (up to 72 hours). The latter attribute is really of benefit only for long sea voyages and spaceflight! Individual variability and visual side effects if use is prolonged are its principal drawbacks.[35] Table 7.1 summarises the leading particulars of some common anti-motion sickness drugs.

Some drug combinations may offer some additional benefit: the primary medication used by astronauts is a combination ("Scop-Dex") of hyoscine and the central sympathomimetic dexamphetamine (in a dose of 0·4 mg and 5 mg respectively) (see also chapter

TABLE 7.1—Leading particulars of some common anti-motion sickness drugs*

Drug	Route of administration	Dose (adult)	Onset of action (h)	Duration of action (h)
Hyoscine	Oral	300–600 µg	0·5	4
	Patch	200 µg + 20 µg h^{-1}	6–8	72
	Injection	200µg	0·25	4
Cinnarizine	Oral	15–30 mg	4	8
Promethazine theoclate	Oral	25 mg	2	24
hydrochloride	Oral	25 mg	2	18
	Injection	50 mg	0·25	18
Dimenhydrinate	Oral	50–100 mg	2	8
Cyclizine	Oral	50 mg	2	12

* After Stott.[32]

12). Dexamphetamine has anti-motion sickness properties of its own, but acts synergistically with promethazine and dimenhydrinate as well as hyoscine.[36] Because dexamphetamine is a controlled substance, the use of this effective combination is unlikely to spread beyond those privileged to be astronauts, but a similar synergism has been demonstrated between ephedrine and both hyoscine and promethazine.[32]

Passengers may also minimise the effects of motion sickness by avoiding anxiety before and during the flight and, when affected, by reducing sensory input by keeping the head as still as possible, preferably by lying down with the eyes shut. This will reduce the intensity of the sickness but not abolish it.

Noise and communication

Noise is essentially a subjective phenomenon and may be regarded as any unwanted sound. It is conveniently expressed on the logarithmic decibel (dB) scale, which allows manageable measurement of the vast range of human hearing, and on which 0 dB is taken as the auditory threshold (equivalent to a sound pressure level of $2 \times 10^{-5} \, N \, m^{-2}$ at a frequency of 1 kHz). A twofold change in noise intensity corresponds to a change in noise level of 3 dB. Normal speech has a level of about 70 dB and a busy street about 80 dB, while high performance military aircraft and helicopters may produce internal noise levels of up to 120 dB.[37] Levels above 125 dB are painful,[38] and rupture of the tympanic membrane occurs at about 160 dB.[39]

Aircraft noise is derived primarily from power sources including transmission systems, propellers (and helicopter rotors), and jet efflux. Noise also emanates from the interaction between the aircraft and the air through which it is moving (boundary layer noise) and from aircraft pressurisation, conditioning, hydraulics, and (most importantly) the communication system itself. The contribution of these various sources to total noise will depend largely on the type of aircraft, phase of flight, and location of the listener. For example the overall noise level inside subsonic jet-powered aircraft usually depends on boundary layer or cabin conditioning noise or both, while outside the aircraft it depends on the jet efflux, especially during takeoff and landing. In helicopters the engine and gearbox transmission, plus the sound of the rotors, provide most internal noise, while the rotor and exhaust produce most external noise.

Noise produces stress in several ways.[40] Above about 90 dB, noise increases the degree of physiological arousal and hence irritability, fatigue, and the risk of accidents. In addition, by masking auditory signals—including speech—high noise levels make many tasks more difficult by increasing the degree of concentration required. The processing of information in active memory is also affected, which increases workload even further.

In the long term, the mechanism of hearing may be damaged, at first reversibly but later permanently. Prolongation of the time taken to recover the temporary threshold shift is an indication that cochleal damage is occurring.[41]

The reduction of both internal and external noise is clearly desirable. In aircraft the development of high bypass ratio jet engines has substantially reduced noise levels, while other more simple approaches—such as increasing canopy thickness, insulating cabin walls, and removing unnecessary airframe protuberances—have reduced aerodynamic noise. The careful siting of new homes, new airports, and flight paths, the restriction of night flying, and adequate home insulation also help reduce the problem.

The noise levels in aircraft inhibit communication both within the aircraft itself and between it and the outside world (air-to-air and air-to-ground). Speech is the only form of communication readily available to aircrew because gesticulation and facial expressions are either inconvenient or impossible. Because speech has great variability in its power spectrum—the consonants having little vocal energy and the vowels much—its integrity needs to be preserved and protected in the face of competing, unwanted sounds. Consequently, special alphabets and methods of pronunciation have been developed in aviation which allow trained speakers to improve their intelligibility substantially.[41] Shouting or increasing the gain of the system both merely raise the overall noise level. Microphones and ear pieces improve communication by attenuating cockpit noise as much as possible, and the efficiency of these devices is usually measured by their ability to maintain intelligibility at low signal-to-noise ratios. A difference of 10–15 dB in speech level over noise will ensure adequate intelligibility of speech and sets the upper limit of acceptable ambient noise at about 85 dB.[41]

Touch and smell

Touch is exploited in aviation in the design and shape of cockpit controls for easy location and recognition. Furthermore, the feedback of tactile sensation (feel) from the controls is of great value to the pilot, although it may be degraded (as in military aviation) if protective gloves have to be worn. Touch may be used as a warning mechanism in future cockpit design, for example by enabling part of the control column to extend to stimulate touch receptors and attract the pilot's attention. Such tactile warning systems in the form of "stick shakers"—which shake the control column violently to warn of impending stall—are already fitted in many aircraft.

Finally, smell is a first-line warning system, indicating fumes within the cabin or, in the case of military aircraft using personal oxygen equipment, suspected contamination of the oxygen supply.

Conclusion

Much of what has been described above is self evident and immutable and there is little that pilots, or their medical advisers, may do to overcome the limitations imposed by flight on human sensory physiology other than to be aware of them. Forewarning will help to forearm.

1 Krefft S. Safety in the air. In: *Folia traumatologica geigy*. Basel: Ciba-Geigy, 1974: 7.
2 Brennan DH. Vision in flight. In: Ernsting J, King PF, eds. *Aviation medicine*, 2nd edn. London: Butterworths, 1988: 346.
3 Curtis JL. Visual problems of high altitude flight. In: Mercier A, ed. *Visual problems in aviation medicine*. Oxford: Pergamon Press, 1962: 39–44.
4 Whiteside TCD. *The problems of vision in flight at high altitude*. London: Butterworths, 1957: 113.
5 Rushton WAH. Visual adaptation. *Proc R Soc Lond (Biol)* 1965; **162:** 20–46.
6 Aircraft instrument and cockpit lighting by red or white light. *Advisory Group for Aerospace Research and Development conference proceedings*. Paris: NATO AGARD, 1967. (AGARD CP-26:iii.)
7 Benson AJ, Burchard E. *Spatial disorientation in flight—a handbook for aircrew*. Neuilly-sur-Seine, France: NATO Advisory Group for Aerospace Research and Development, 1973. (AGARDograph No 170.)
8 Benson AJ. Spatial disorientation—general aspects. In: Ernsting J, King PF, eds. *Aviation medicine*, 2nd edn. London: Butterworths, 1988: 279.
9 Lyons TJ, Ercoline WR, Freeman JE, Gillingham KK. Epidemiology of USAF spatial disorientation accidents from 1989–1991. *Aviat Space Environ Med* 1993; **64** (in press).
10 Lyons TJ, Harding RM, Freeman JE, Oakley C. G-induced loss of consciousness accidents: USAF experience 1982–1990. *Aviat Space Environ Med* 1992; **63:** 60–6.
11 Vyrnwy-Jones P. A review of army air corps helicopter accidents. *Aviat Space Environ Med* 1985; **56:** 403–9.
12 Vyrnwy-Jones P. *Disorientation accidents and incidents in US army helicopters*. US Army Aeromedical Research Laboratory, Fort Rucker, 1988; Report No 88–3.
13 Kirkham WR, Collins WE, Grape PM, Simpson JM, Wallace TF. Spatial disorientation in general aviation accidents. *Aviat Space Environ Med* 1978; **49:** 1080–6.

14 Civil Aviation Authority. Visual flight rules. In: *United Kingdom air pilot, Vol. 1*. London: CAA, 1975 (as amended).

15 Civil Aviation Authority. *Reportable accidents to UK registered aircraft, and to foreign registered aircraft in UK airspace, 1990*. London: CAA CAP 600, 1992: 115.

16 Benson AJ. Spatial disorientation—common illusions. In: Ernsting J, King PF, eds. *Aviation medicine*, 2nd edn. London: Butterworths, 1988: 302.

17 Graybiel A, Hupp DI. The oculogyral illusion. *J Aviat Med* 1946; **17:** 3–27.

18 Gillingham KK, Krutz RW. Effects of the abnormal acceleratory environment of flight. *Aeromed Rev* 1974: **10:**74.

19 Wicks RE. Alternobaric vertigo: an aeromedical review. *Aviat Space Environ Med* 1966; **60:** 67–72.

20 Benson AJ. Spatial disorientation and the "break-off" phenomenon. *Aerospace Med* 1973; **44:** 944–52.

21 Edgington K, Box CJ. Disorientation in army helicopter operations. *J Soc Occup Med* 1982; **32:** 128–35.

22 Reason JT. *Man in motion—the psychology of travel*. London: Weidenfeld and Nicolson, 1974: 26–37.

23 Treisman M. Motion sickness: an evolutionary hypothesis. *Science* 1977; **197:** 493–5.

24 Money KE, Cheung BS. Another function of the inner ear: facilitation of the emetic response to poisons. *Aviat Space Environ Med* 1983; **54:** 208–11.

25 Money KE. Motion sickness and evolution. In: Crampton GH, ed. *Motion and space sickness*. Boca Raton, FL: CRC Press, 1989: 1–7.

26 Money KE. Simulator sickness and its basic nature. In: *Motion sickness: significance in aerospace operations and prophylaxis*. Neuilly-sur-Seine, France: NATO Advisory Group for Aerospace Research and Development, 1991; AGARD LS-175: 6B.1–6B.4.

27 Rubin HJ. Air sickness in a primary air force training detachment. *Aviat Med* 1942; **13:** 272.

28 Dobie TG. *Air sickness in aircrew*. Neuilly-sur-Seine, France: NATO Advisory Group for Aerospace Research and Development, 1974. (AGARDograph AG-177.)

29 Hixon WC, Guedry FE, Lentz JM. Results of a longitudinal study of airsickness incidence during naval flight officer training. In: *Motion sickness: mechanisms, prediction, prevention and treatment*. Neuilly-sur-Seine, France: NATO Advisory Group for Aerospace Research and Development, 1984; AGARD CP-372: 30.1–30.13.

30 Benson AJ. Motion sickness. In: Ernsting J, King PF, eds. *Aviation medicine*, 2nd edn. London: Butterworths, 1988: 329.

31 Bagshaw M, Stott JRR. The desensitisation of chronically motion sick aircrew in the Royal Air Force. *Aviat Space Environ Med* 1985; **56:** 1144–51.

32 Stott JRR. Management of acute and chronic motion sickness. In: *Motion sickness: significance in aerospace operations and prophylaxis*. Neuilly-sur-Seine, France: NATO Advisory Group for Aerospace Research and Development, 1991; AGARD LS-175: 11.1–11.7.

33 Hargreaves J. The prophylaxis of seasickness—a comparison of cinnarizine with hyoscine. *Practitioner* 1982; **226:** 160.

34 Pingree BJW, Pethybridge RJ. A double-blind placebo controlled comparison of hyoscine with early administered cinnarizine in increasing tolerance to a nauseogenic cross-coupled stimulus. *Pharm Med* 1989; **4:** 29–42.

35 Parrott AC. Transdermal scopolamine: a review of its effects upon motion sickness, psychological performance, and physiological functioning. *Aviat Space Environ Med* 1989; **60:** 1–9.

36 Wood CD. Pharmacological countermeasures against motion sickness. In: Crampton GH, ed. *Motion and space sickness*. Boca Raton, FL: CRC Press, 1989: 343–51.

37 Green RG. Noise and communication. In: Dhenin G, ed. *Aviation medicine*, Vol 1. London: Tri-Med Books, 1978: 528.

38 Ades HW, Merrill SN, Graybiel A, Tolhurst GC. Threshold of aural pain to high intensity sound. *Aerospace Med* 1959; **30:** 678–84.

39 Parrack HO. Effects of acoustic energy. In: Armstrong HG, ed. *Aerospace medicine*. London: Baillière, Tindall and Cox, 1961: 294.

40 Poulton EC. Blue collar stressors. In: Cooper CL, Paybe R, eds. *Stress at work*. Chichester: John Wiley & Sons, 1978: 55–8.

41 Green RG. Auditory communication. In: Nicholson AN, ed. *Fourth advanced operational aviation medicine course*. Report No 642. Neuilly-sur-Seine, France: NATO Advisory Group for Aerospace Research and Development, 1976: 25–7.

8
Aviation psychology

I am a brother to dragons and a companion to owls.[1]

In research into human factors in aviation the respective roles of the psychologist and doctor are not well demarcated, and in recognition of this indistinct borderline this chapter on aviation psychology has been included. To some extent, however, aviation psychology is an entire and separate pursuit, so what follows can provide only an impression of the scope and nature of the subject.

Perceptual limitations

Many psychological problems have been referred to in previous chapters—for example, vestibular illusions and communication in noise, both of which are as much of psychological as of medical interest. A further problem is the way in which pilots use visual cues, particularly in the approach to land. Pilots are unlikely to be able to identify the cues which they use during the approach (fig 8.1) because, as with many skills, it is not necessary to be able to describe the components of that skill in order to possess it.

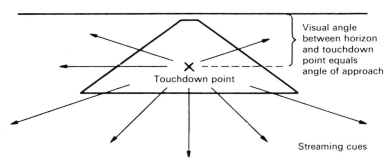

FIG 8.1—Schematic representation of runway shape, visual angle, and streaming cues.

Nevertheless, with thought and experiment the possible cues available to the pilot may be identified, namely the way in which the world appears to stream past the viewer, the textural gradient in the terrain, the visual angle between the horizon and the touchdown point (that is, the angle of approach, the projected shape of the runway on the retina, and possibly some others).[2,3] Individual pilots probably do not use all available cues but unconsciously attend only to an idiosyncratic subset which is found to be adequate during training.[4] Thus, if on an approach where special circumstances have removed or altered a cue which is important to a particular pilot—for example if snow cover has hidden the texture of the terrain—he or she may have difficulty when another pilot does not. The shape of the runway may present a similar problem. A pilot who relies on the perceived shape of the runway may be misled by an abnormally long runway which will appear to be the same shape as a shorter one viewed from a shallower angle of approach. Errors such as these may induce the pilot to land either long (some distance down the runway from its threshold) or short (before the runway threshold); the latter is usually the less desirable.

Midair collisions are also of interest to the psychologist of vision.[5] If two aircraft at constant speeds and on constant headings are going to collide then they maintain constant relative bearings to one another (fig 8.2); all other aircraft will possess some relative motion. This means that the aircraft which it is most important for the pilot to detect appears stationary on the windscreen, and the small amount of movement to which the peripheral retina is so sensitive is completely absent. The aircraft is also unlikely to be detected because its size stays very small on the retina until shortly before collision (fig 8.3), and detection thus relies on efficient visual search by the pilot. The small size of the target requires that it must be detected foveally, or near foveally, and the discontinuous saccadic nature of visual search makes detection only probable.[6] Thus, unfortunately, the combination of physical, physiological, and psychological circumstances makes the detection of an aircraft on a collision course less likely than that of an aircraft which poses no such threat, and extensive field trials have shown that the likelihood of a collision being avoided because of target acquisition is surprisingly low.[7] A pilot detecting an aircraft shortly before a potential collision may avoid it if he or she can react quickly enough. Despite the fact that much is made by the

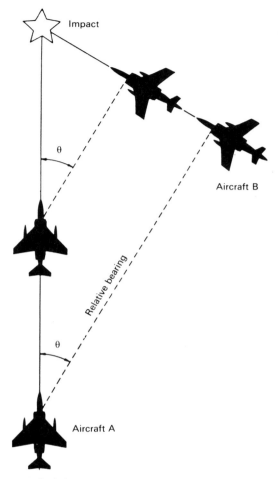

Impact

θ

Aircraft B

Relative bearing

θ

Aircraft A

FIG 8.2—Constancy of relative bearings for aircraft on collision courses.

layperson of the quick reactions of pilots, fast responses are rarely required in flight. The pilot is almost always best advised to consider a decision rather than to respond in haste. Two specific accidents in which fast responses were required[8,9] have, however, led to experimental work in simulators, which indicates that the sort of simple response times found in the psychological laboratory[10] give little guidance to the applied psychologist. When pilots

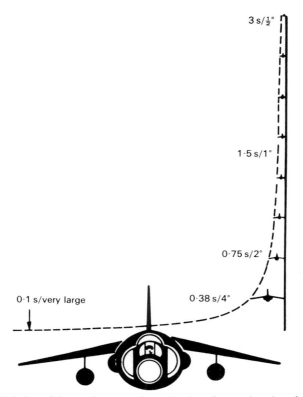

FIG 8.3—Relation of time to impact and angular size of oncoming aircraft.

are presented with unexpected emergencies their response times are long and variable, from 2 to perhaps 7 s.[8] Such long response times are determined not by the time required to make the response but by the time required for the pilot to grasp an unusual, unexpected, or complex event—the so called cognition time. To the designer of a terrain-following autopilot, which relies on the pilot to intervene and prevent the aircraft striking the ground in the event of a system failure, this fact may be unpalatable but it is inescapable. This is one respect in which the design must accommodate the person rather than vice versa—a principle which is central to the specialty known as engineering psychology or, more broadly, ergonomics.

105

Problems of equipment

Displays

Reference to the increasing complexity of aircraft instrument displays since the first world war has become an aviation cliché. Interpreting apparently complicated instrument arrays is, however, not as difficult as it first appears because only a limited subset of instruments requires constant or regular attention and many need monitoring only in certain phases of flight. The experienced pilot is also accustomed to the patterns of display presented by instruments (their arrangement being designed to facilitate this) and should quickly be able to identify a deviation from normal. Despite this, problems with displays and controls arise with depressing regularity.

The best known problem is that of the "three pointer altimeter". Aircraft instruments have traditionally been designed as circular dials with indicator needles, and some early altimeters resembled clocks in having a stubby needle which indicated thousands of feet and a slim needle which indicated the remaining hundreds of feet. As aircraft flew higher the display of tens of thousands of feet was needed, and a new, very stubby, needle was added (fig 8.4). The unwitting lethality incorporated in such instruments was highlighted in 1958, when in two separate incidents Viscount and Britannia airliners flew into the ground after their pilots had reported their altitudes to air traffic controllers as being 3048 m (10 000 ft) higher than they actually were.[11,12] It is easy to misread instruments designed like this, for the most important pointer is

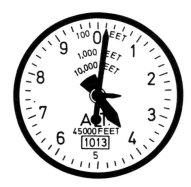

FIG 8.4—A three pointer altimeter.

the smallest and hence the easiest to misapprehend.[13] This particular problem is easily solved by the provision of a counter, or digital readout, on the altimeter (although many aircraft flying today still have three pointer instruments), yet this does not represent a general case for greater use of digital instruments. Many displays, such as fuel gauges, are best presented with an analogue component to the display. It is much easier for a busy pilot to assess his fuel state by looking at the position of a needle on a gauge than by reading the number of remaining kilos; since for the latter he must mentally refer the observed digital value to the memorised values of maximum capacity and minimum permissible level.

The invasion of the modern cockpit by electronic displays[14,15] has placed enormous demands on the engineering psychologist. In modern military and civil aircraft, multifunction cathode ray tubes have replaced many of the conventional instruments. The potential of these displays—to present information only when it is required and in colour, to overlay radar returns on a moving map, and to display check lists and lists of emergency actions—is enormous. All of these possibilities must be carefully evaluated to ensure that some reincarnation of the three pointer altimeter is not being unintentionally designed into these systems. Perhaps the main difference between electronic displays and traditional instruments is the capacity of the former to present widely differing information on the same display surface. The consequence of this is that unlike conventional instrumentation not all information is displayed constantly. Heavy reliance must be placed on the computers, which decide when the pilot needs to be warned of an incipient or actual system failure. This, in turn, places an onerous load on the designer to anticipate all possible combinations of such failure.

Presenting the pilot with a well integrated display that combines complex data to provide a relatively simple and clear picture of the aircraft's situation also means that the pilot is no longer in a good position to question the accuracy of the displays, which can lead to the phenomenon known as 'over-trust'. The control and display systems of such aircraft are invariably highly computerised, making a large range of control and display options or modes available to the pilot, and several accidents have occurred due to failures of pilot 'mode awareness' (that is, the pilot believed that he had programmed the aircraft to behave in a different way from that actually programmed).

Such difficulties must be resolved if the relationship between the pilot and the systems of automated aircraft are to be successful.

Warning systems

With a wide variety but low actual incidence of possible failures there is a temptation to warn the pilot by associating each fault with an auditory signal. The hazards of such practice are illustrated by the (apocryphal) story of the pilot who landed without lowering his undercarriage, although air traffic control was warning him by radio. He later explained that he could not hear them because his aircraft had been fitted with a klaxon to warn that the undercarriage had not been lowered. The problem of abstract tones with no inherent meaning is exacerbated in modern aircraft, in which navigational and warning tones are numerous.

Warning displays must, of course, be reliable. All large British commercial aircraft are fitted with a ground proximity warning system. The difficulty of triggering such a warning system reliably resulted in frequent false alarms, and pilots became familiar with the noise—a familiarity which bred sufficient contempt for several aircraft to be flown into the ground with the warning sounding. Of the 43 fatal accidents to worldwide commercial aircraft during 1992 (excluding sabotage), "controlled flight into terrain" was declared the cause in 21, and claimed the lives of 706 people.[16]

Controls

Displays represent only one half of the interface between pilot and machine: the pilot must also control the aircraft, and this represents another rapidly changing topic of interest for the engineering psychologist. Although the control column and throttle controls of many current aircraft are still familiar, some new factors are dictating the necessity for change. The next generation of fighter aircraft will include highly advanced computer controlled aerodynamic surfaces. The pilot will not demand a control surface deflection but a manoeuvre; the computer will then decide how best to produce that manoeuvre given the state of many variables including speed, angle of attack, weight, centre of gravity, and altitude. With such sophistication, new types of canard control can be contemplated that will allow direct horizontal and vertical translational forces to be developed on the airframe so that, for example, the aircraft may gain height without any rotation in pitch. Precisely how the pilot will demand these extra dimensions of control remains to be discovered.

Some current civil aircraft have already dispensed with any 'hard' linkage between the pilot's control and the control surfaces: the link is made only via electronic signalling and sophisticated computing. This can provide many benefits, not least in preventing the pilot from placing the aircraft outside the 'envelope' in which it is designed to fly, but the requirements for such control systems to operate in a completely error free way are obvious.

Workload

The principal impact on the crew of improved technology on the flight deck has been a reduction in the number of tasks that the crew must perform, but an increase in the amount of information that must be monitored. Under such circumstances it is difficult to determine the extent of the pilot's workload, yet its assessment is crucial in deciding how many people are required to operate a given aircraft. In a military interceptor the benefits of having an additional person on board may be offset by the extra weight and performance penalties that the extra person entails. Airline economics dictate the presence of only the minimum number of flight crew commensurate with safe operation, and in a modern airliner only two people are present on the flight deck. These matters are overlaid with so many politicoindustrial considerations that an objective means of assessing workload is clearly desirable. Indeed the "two v three" crew issue was so strongly debated in the United States that a president's task force on crew complement was set up.[17] The report of this committee has stimulated the Federal Aviation Administration to insist that workload has been formally assessed on any new aircraft before it will be certificated. It does not, however, answer the psychologist's problem of how to carry out such an assessment. Many techniques have been suggested, but these resolve themselves into methods that require the aircrew to give some form of rating of how hard they feel themselves to be working (the most famous of these being the Cooper–Harper scale[18]), secondary task techniques,[19] observational techniques in which the overt activity of the aircrew is analysed,[20] and the measurement of physiological variables, principally heart rate.[21]

All of these methods have severe deficiencies: subjective ratings are open to subjective bias, secondary tasks are intrusive, observation cannot indicate the cognitive load on the pilot, and heart rate is more affected by the pilot's perception of how critical the task is than by how complex the task is. Aircraft seeking certification in the United States have to use some combination of the techniques described above, but there is some encouraging basic psychological research (looking at ways of assessing how finite mental resources can be allocated) that may yield more acceptable methods of measuring workload.[22-24]

Social relationships

A critical factor in aircraft safety is the way in which individual members of a crew relate to one another. The importance of such social interactions should not be overlooked because in many accidents failure of communication between crew members, or failure of the captain to make the fullest use of the expertise of other crew members, has been cited as material factors. In some accidents, breakdown of communication between flight deck and cabin crew members have had disastrous consequences as, for example, when the cabin crew have seen an engine on fire but remained unaware that the flight deck crew was wrongly shutting down the functioning engine.

Many changes to the way pilots are trained have been made in an attempt to combat such problems, but the major emphasis is on training crews as teams rather than as individuals. This has represented a considerable change of approach in an area where training, licensing, and checking had always been carried out on an individual rather than a group basis.

The ways in which members of a group interact are complex, because they depend (on the flight deck) on the role, status, personality, and ability of each team member. Given the importance of this problem, it may be predicted with some confidence that research into the social or group aspects of aircrew performance will be of future importance.

Personality and selection

At the moment there is no formal method of identifying and selecting potential pilots with respect to their personality. Indeed, the method of selection used by the Royal Air Force has changed little since the war:[25] it (and most airlines) rely on interviews and other subjective means to assess the character or personality of recruits. Not only does the personality of potential pilots need to be assessed, however, but also their aptitude to perform the task. Considerable psychological research has been carried out into aptitude testing in aviation but it has had disappointing results. The main reason for any selection system is, of course, to save time and money. It would be quite feasible to use flying training itself as a selection process, allowing all candidates to start training and gradually eliminating those who fail to cope. In a system where the number of aircraft available is typically less than one tenth of the number of those volunteering to fly, however, some selection at the beginning is required. The usual procedure in any selection system is to analyse the job, to attempt to identify the skills required, to devise a set of scorable tasks that use those skills, and then to validate the tasks by computing the level of correlation between the score on the tasks and the trainee's final level of flying competence or likelihood of completing training—the criterion score. This is illustrated in fig 8.5: typical individual correlation coefficients in selection for flying are fairly low, and the individual data points may be enclosed by an ellipse of the type shown. Section (a) represents those who passed the selection test and passed flying training and section (b) those who passed selection but failed flying training. Research on this topic is hampered by the fact that full information on the shape of this figure is unobtainable because as

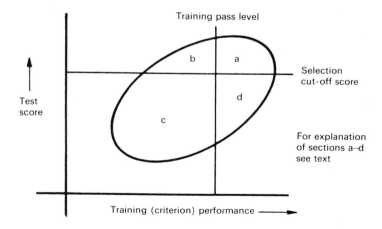

FIG 8.5—Relation between selection test and training performances.

soon as a candidate fails the selection test no further data are available. Thus the precise nature of areas (c) and especially (d) (the test failures who would have passed the course) cannot be known in a working system. In practice, several aptitude tests are used, individually assessed, and then weighted in proportion to efficacy before being summed to generate a pilot index.[26] In the Royal Air Force today these selection techniques are augmented by a short period of formal flying training, when further selection is made.

Another intractable difficulty in designing a selection process is in the very first step of analysing the skills requirement of the job. Aircraft in the second world war required a high level of psychomotor coordination from the pilot, and the present selection tests still reflect this. Today's pilot must also possess such skills but, more importantly, should be able to assess quickly the priorities of the components of the task, be able to combine information from various channels to provide a coherent image of events, and have sufficient spare mental resource to be able to think and plan while controlling the aircraft. Traditional techniques of selection do not cover such requirements, but as microcomputers become more flexible and available, selection testing is becoming increasingly sophisticated and soon the first real changes in pilot selection for 40 years will take place.

The types of artificial task used in the selection process are very similar to those used in the laboratory of the psychologist who examines the effects of stress on performance.

Stress, performance, and error

The variety of stresses to which a fighter pilot is subjected is probably wider than for any other occupation. The effects on performance of these physical and mental stresses—heat, noise, acceleration, vibration, hypoxia, anxiety, sleep deprivation, and fatigue—have already been referred to in previous chapters and are well reviewed elsewhere.[27] Theoretical models also exist for the effects of stress on performance.[28,29] The relevance of all this work to the definition of the cockpit environment is critical. For example, the larger the pressure differential that the aircraft hull must maintain the greater will be its weight and cost: thus strong economic influences exist to maximise the cabin altitude of aircraft. Care must be taken, however, to maintain the physiology and psychology of the inhabitants: the more stringent of these two requirements is the maintenance of psychological function. Experimental studies have shown effects of hypoxia on performance at altitudes as low as 1525 m (5000 ft),[30] but recent work highlights how fickle and variable such effects on performance may be, making practical interpretation of results extremely difficult.[31,32] The same is true of the effects of heat on performance: some workers have reported improvements in performance with increasing heat[32] while others have detected decrements.[33] What is clear is that even an apparently simple stress, such as heat, will produce different effects on performance depending on the subject's relative skin and core temperatures and whether he or she is being heated or cooled.

Although it is difficult to model the effects of many such stresses on performance, a deterministic understanding will probably eventually be reached. There is, however, a large area of research into stress that is even more difficult—that of so called life stress. It seems intuitively reasonable that the performance of a pilot who has serious domestic problems might be affected. Much research has taken place in this area over the past decade,[34] and there is some evidence of a relation between the amount of life stress or life change experienced and the likelihood of illness.[35] Some research has also aimed at testing the hypothesis that those pilots who experience more than normal life change will also have a greater than normal chance of being in a flying accident, perhaps because of their preoccupation with their non-flying problems. Individual case studies tend to support such a notion, but statistical population studies do not provide any corroboration,[36] possibly because life stress is just one of the many features that may be important in the aetiology of accidents due to "human factors". The limitations of human sensory function, the design of displays and controls, and the social relationships on the flight deck are all of obvious importance, and it is true to say that all the effort of the civil aviation psychologist is ultimately aimed at preventing accidents.

The specific study of error has always concerned the most eminent psychologists,[37,38] and the importance of preventing accidents not only in aircraft but also in, for example, nuclear power stations has added new urgency to the problem. In the search for the "accident prone" several studies have shown that the neurotic extravert is more likely to be involved in a driving accident than the stable introvert[39] and that those identified in questionnaire studies as "adventurous" have a much greater probability of being involved in a flying accident.[40] Characteristically, the "adventurous" personality is likely to be involved in an accident as a result of illegal low flying. It is the delicate task of the air force commander to encourage legally aggressive flying but to contain excessive risk taking or rule breaking by the few. The problem, of course, is to identify who the few are: individuals continually role play, and the flying supervisor may not identify a risk taking individual during normal contact. Assessing pilots more formally in this respect may thus help to identify suspect pilots and improve their management.

A more detailed understanding of the sort of lapses that occur to us all (that is, doing one thing when another was intended) may be of even greater benefit. Many flying accidents occur because the pilot makes the (correct) decision to operate a particular control but in fact operates another. Examples of this behaviour are legion, but they attract most attention when spectacular consequences arise, such as when a pilot shuts a fuel cock when he intended to manipulate the cabin heater or when on the ground he intended to raise the canopy but in fact raised the undercarriage. Better ergonomics might help to overcome this problem, but a fuller understanding of the underlying mechanisms of human skills is a prerequisite of solution, if indeed solution is possible.

In the investigation of accidents, however, it is no longer the individual who commits the precipitating error who receives most attention from the investigating team: the organisation of which that individual forms a part is coming under increasing scrutiny. The policies of organisations are being questioned to ensure that safety has received adequate recognition at the highest level of management in all of the company's operations. This is not being done simply to avoid the unfairness of a pilot being blamed for a mistake that was at least partially engendered by poor operational rules or equipment, but because blaming the individual does little to avoid the possibility of recurrence, whereas changing an underlying cause can reap future safety benefits.

Conclusion

In this brief survey of aviation psychology no mention has been made of some other important topics such as training and checking pilots, and the psychosocial problems of alcohol and flying. Nevertheless, we hope that some insight has been given to its scope, and to the important part played by the psychologist in many facets of aviation.

1 Job XXX, 29. *Holy Bible*, King James version.
2 Gibson JJ. *The perception of the visual world*. London: Allen and Unwin, 1952.
3 Mertens HW. Perception of runway image shape and approach angle magnitude by pilots in simulated night landing approaches. *Aviat Space Environ Med* 1981; **52:** 373–86.
4 Chappelow JW, Smart JA. Putting texture in perspective. *Proceedings of the Royal Aeronautical Society's two day flight simulation symposium*. London: Royal Aeronautical Society, 1982: 1–6.
5 Green RG. Mid air collisions—how to avoid them. *Air Clues* 1982; **July:** 260–2.
6 Harris JL. Visual aspects of air collision. In: *Visual search—proceedings of the 1970 annual symposium of the committee on vision*. Washington DC: National Academy of Sciences, 1973: 26–50.
7 Andrews JW. *Air-to-air visual acquisition performance with TCAS II*. Lexington, MA: Lincoln Laboratory, 1984. (MIT Report No DOT/FAA/PM-84/17.)
8 Green RG, Skinner R. Response times to locked controls at rotation. In: *Report on the accident to BAe HS 748 G-BEKF at Sumburgh Airport, Shetland Islands on 31 July 1979*. London: Department of Trade, 1981. (Department of Trade Accidents Investigation Branch Report 1/81.)
9 Chappelow JW. An investigation of the time taken to respond to total engine failure. In: *Report on the accident to Wessex 60 GAS WI at 52°56'N 01°46'E*. London: Department of Trade.
10 Kling JW, Riggs LA. *Woodworth and Schlosberg's experimental psychology*. New York: Holt, Rinehart and Winston, 1971.
11 Civil Aviation Authority. *Report on the accident to Viscount type 802 G-AORC which occurred on 28th April 1958, at Tarbolton, Ayrshire*. London: Civil Aviation Authority 1959: CAP 154. (Civil Accident Report C679.)
12 Civil Aviation Authority. *Report on the accident to Britannia G-AOVD which occurred on 24th December 1958, at Sopley Park, Christchurch, Hants*. London: Civil Aviation Authority 1960: CAP 164. (Civil Accident Report C693.)
13 Rolfe JM. Human factors and the display of height information. *Appl Ergon* 1969; **1:** 70.
14 Stonehouse D. Evolution of the airborne display. *Electr Eng* 1980; **52:** 29–45.
15 Howell GC. The modern military aircraft cockpit. *Electr Eng* 1980; **52:** 47–55.
16 Learmount D. Not under control. *Flight International* 1993; **143** (Number 4354): 27–34.
17 McLucas JL, Drinkwater FJ, Leaf HW. *Report of the President's task force on aircraft crew complement*. Washington, DC: US State Department, 1981.
18 Cooper GE, Harper RP. *The use of pilot rating in the evaluation of aircraft handling qualities*. Washington, DC: NASA, 1969. (Technical Note 5153.)
19 Green R, Flux R. Auditory communication and workload. In: *Methods to assess workload*. Neuilly-sur-Seine, France: NATO Advisory Group for Aerospace Research and Development, 1978: A4.1–A4.8 (AGARD Conference Proceedings No 216).
20 Chiles WD. *Objective methods for developing indices of pilot workload*. Washington, DC: Federal Aviation Authority. FA-AM-77-15, 1977.
21 Roscoe AH. Handling qualities, workload and heart rate. In: Hartman BO, McKenzie RE, eds. *Survey of methods to assess workload*. Neuilly-sur-Seine, France: NATO Advisory Group for Aerospace Research and Development, 1979. (AGARD No 246.)
22 Norman DA, Bobrow DG. On data-limited and resource-limited processes. *Cogn Psychol* 1975; **7:** 44–64.
23 Norman DA, Bobrow DG. On the analysis of performance operating characteristics. *Psychol Rev* 1976; **83:** 508–10.
24 Broadbent DE. Task combination and selective intake of information. *Acta Psychol* 1982; **83:** 253–90.
25 Vernon PE, Parry JB. *Personnel selection in British armed forces*. London: London University Press, 1949: 67–82.
26 Knight S. Validation of RAF pilot selection measures. *Note for the record No 7178*. London: Ministry of Defence, 1978.
27 Poulton EC. *Environment and human efficiency*. Springfield, IL: Thomas, 1970.
28 Broadbent DE. *Decision and stress*. London: Academic Press, 1971.

29 Warburton DM, Hamilton V, eds. *Human stress and cognition—an information processing approach*. New York: John Wiley & Sons, 1979.
30 Denison DM, Ledwith F, Poulton EC. Complex reaction times at simulated altitudes of 5000 feet and 8000 feet. *Aerospace Med* 1966; **37:** 1010–13.
31 Green RG, Morgan DR. Effects of mild hypoxia on a logical reasoning task. *Preprints of the 54th annual scientific meeting of the Aerospace Medical Association*. Washington, DC: Aerospace Medical Association 1983: 194–5.
32 Poulton EC. Arousing environmental stresses can improve performance whatever people say. *Aviat Space Environ Med* 1976; **47:** 1193–204.
33 Allen JR, Gibson TM, Green RG. Effect of induced cyclic changes of deep body temperature on task performances. *Aviat Space Environ Med* 1979; **50:** 585–9.
34 Johnson JH, Sarason IG. Recent developments in life stress. In: Warburton DM, Hamilton V, eds. *Human stress and cognition—an information processing approach*. New York: John Wiley & Sons, 1979: 205–33.
35 Rahe RH, Arthur RJ. Life change and illness studies—past history and future directions. *J Hum Stress* 1978; **4:** 3–15.
36 Alkov RA, Borowsky MS. A questionnaire study of psychological background factors in US navy aircraft accidents. *Aviat Space Environ Med* 1980; **51:** 860–3.
37 Freud S. *The psychopathology of everyday life*. London: Ernest Benn Ltd, 1914.
38 James W. *The principles of psychology. Vol 1*. New York: Henry Holt and Company, 1890.
39 Shaw L, Sichel H. *Accident proneness*. Oxford: Pergamon Press, 1971.
40 Levine JB, Lee JO, Ryman DH, Rahe RH. Attitudes and accidents aboard an aircraft carrier. *Aviat Space Environ Med* 1976; **47:** 82–5.

9

Medical aspects of airline operations

... the whole civil aviation industry is working to one end, namely the safe passage of an aircraft through a physiologically and physically hostile environment.[1]

On 25 August 1919 the first British regular scheduled international commercial air service began between London and Paris. That year also saw the inauguration of commercial aviation in France, Germany, and the United States. The growth of civil aviation has been such that the world's airlines made 1·125 billion passenger journeys on scheduled services during 1991.[2] Because of security fears, this figure was less than that for 1990 (1·16 billion) but 1992 saw a return to the previous upward trend in scheduled international traffic, which increased by about 13%. This chapter deals with some of the medical aspects of supporting such a vast industry, both in the air and on the ground.

Commercial aircraft must be so designed, constructed, and managed that they meet the myriad national and international regulations governing every aspect of their use. Many of these regulations are of an engineering, technological, or administrative nature, but there are several areas, covering both routine and emergency operations, which are legitimately the concern of doctors in general and aviation medicine specialists in particular.

Hygiene

The wellbeing and safety of everyone on board commercial aircraft may be seriously compromised if insufficient attention is paid to routine matters of health and hygiene. This would be most obvious if, for example, an entire crew was stricken by acute gastroenteritis:[3] hence the sound and widely followed advice to

117

pilots that they should eat different dishes not only while on board the aircraft but also in hotels and restaurants before a flight.[4] Less obvious, perhaps, are the dangers inherent in poor airport sanitation arrangements whereby food may be easily contaminated or waste may attract scavengers.

Catering

Airline catering is an enormous and daunting undertaking. British Airways alone serves nearly 24 million meals to passengers each year from some 160 stations located in all parts of the globe: over 12 million meals originate in London alone. Catering must therefore be of the highest hygienic standard so that food poisoning—and particularly the ubiquitous salmonellosis—is avoided. Careful control over the food itself, the food handlers, and the premises in which food is prepared is essential.[5] Airlines prefer to supply and prepare food in their own kitchens, where control is easier, but this is not always possible. Kitchens operated by subcontractors must be supervised by the airlines (or, in the case of airport catering facilities, by the airport authority), and if this is not feasible then the right of inspection and batch sampling must be retained and implemented. Catering staff should undergo strict medical examinations before employment and be re-examined regularly thereafter; continuing instruction in food handling and hygiene should be encouraged. In the United Kingdom, premises where food is prepared are governed by the Food Safety Act 1990, an enabling act which allows regulations concerning the handling and storage of food, and other measures such as the use of bactericidal hand cleaners, of hot water rinses, and of disposable hats and gloves to be imposed and updated as needed.[6] The Food Safety Act also calls for suitable mandatory training of food handlers, but neglects to state what "suitable" means—the United Kingdom airline industry has therefore taken upon itself the development of a code of practice for its caterers, and has also instituted an inflight food hygiene code of practice, and enhanced food hygiene training for senior staff. The risks associated with certain foodstuffs (including poultry, shellfish, cold meat, cheeses, and fresh cream) must be minimised. For the first time, water was classified as a food by the 1990 act. If food is not to be consumed immediately the requirements for storage must be rigorously enforced: cold foods must be stored below 8°C while hot food must be stored above 63°C.[56] This is particularly important if the airline practices "double" or "return" catering, where food for both outward and return flights is supplied by the parent airport.

Aircraft are not always able to carry sufficient drinking water for a round trip and may have to "top up" during ground stops. All airports must therefore have a supply of pure water, which is palatable and free from colour, odour, and turbidity, together with a safe means of delivering it to aircraft.[7] Once on board, drinking water may be supplied from small independent sources while other needs are met from a separate supply. Usually (and preferably), however, because of the risk of contamination, all water on a large aircraft is of drinkable quality and is supplied from large steel or fibreglass tanks. A single aircraft may have "topped up" from several places during a long trip and so the WHO recommends that, however reliable a source may be, all supplies should be effectively chlorinated immediately before being loaded on the aircraft:[5] this is usually carried out in the airport water bowsers. Dechlorination before drinking is then necessary to ensure palatability; taste neutralising tablets are added by the crew after water has been drawn from the tanks. Micropore filters, whose primary function is to help neutralise chlorine, are fitted at all water inlets in some aircraft but may be a contamination hazard themselves unless they are changed regularly. All waste water is drained overboard and not held for later disposal. The possibility of atmospheric pollution by contaminated waste water has led to the suggestion that isolated and otherwise unexplained outbreaks of cholera in places underlying air routes from India and the middle east may be due to infected effluent from overflying aircraft.[8]

Sanitation

Aircraft toilets, ideally numbering at least one per 25 passengers on long range aircraft, are essentially chemical closets which empty into retention tanks. (The ideal ratio is very optimistic: British Airways aims at one toilet per 32 passengers on long range aircraft while most short haul aircraft have one per 50 passengers.) The flushing mechanism is usually electric. Waste material is filtered and part of the liquid phase is recycled for flushing after an appropriate chemical has been added. The chemical additive, often a quaternary ammonium compound (which, while not as effective as the glutaraldehyde used previously, is not a recognised carcinogen) must meet stringent requirements, including consistent and efficient bactericidal and cleansing activity, aesthetic acceptability

119

(odour and colour), and stability: that is, it must be totally effective when correctly diluted. No adequate viricidal agent is currently available and, consequently, the risk to waste handlers of infections such as hepatitis is very real. The solid phase, and any remaining liquid, is held in the retention tank before being discharged after landing, ideally into a main sewer directly from the aircraft or via a toilet waste vehicle. Airports must have a failsafe disposal system and strict control of cleanliness: separation of staff concerned with water supply and waste disposal is essential.

Cabin cleanliness

The state of aircraft interiors is important, not only because of appearance but also for reasons of health, and so all cabin, galley, and toilet areas should be tidied and cleaned thoroughly during each turnround. There must also be suitable arrangements in the galley areas for collection of kitchen waste while in flight.

Cabin air quality

Australia long ago joined Canada, China, Israel, Norway, the then Soviet Union, and Sweden in banning smoking on domestic flights; Canada at least has judged the move to be a commercial success.[9] A similar ban was imposed by the Federal Aviation Administration for domestic flights throughout the United States from April 1988, and by British Airways in the United Kingdom from October of that year.[10] At the time, British Airways was, uniquely and commendably, acting on its own initiative; smoking bans in all the other nations listed being government inspired. It must be said, however, that these moves were possibly not quite as altruistic as at first may appear because they coincided with the need to improve the quality of circulating air in aircraft cabins. Until the late 1980s, 400–600 l of *fresh* air were delivered to the cabin per person per minute. In modern aircraft, this figure has been reduced to 150–180 l per person per minute, although the total requirement remains the same: consequently the rest is *recirculated* air.

Concern about contamination of this recirculating volume with environmental tobacco smoke, and the increased awareness of the health risks associated with passive smoking, was in part responsible for the widespread ban on smoking,[10] although commercial pressure from nonsmoking customers was also relevant. In late 1989, the United States department of transportation commissioned a study (by Geomet Technologies Inc) into environmental tobacco smoke and other potential pollutants of cabin air: carbon dioxide, microbial aerosols, ozone, and cosmic radiation.[11] Levels of all but the last of these substances were measured during 92 randomly selected flights (23 nonsmoking, and 69 smoking). Cosmic radiation was not measured directly because accurate methods exist to forecast its levels; this very important subject is discussed in greater detail in chapter 11. Levels of microbial aerosols never approached those associated with a risk of illness, and ozone levels likewise remained well below the Federal Aviation Administration's 3-hour standard of 0·10 ppm (although other studies have shown levels well in excess of the standard). Ozone is also considered in greater detail in chapter 11. Carbon dioxide levels are used as an indication of efficiency of ventilation: as the fresh air component declines so the CO_2 level may be expected to rise. Not surprisingly, therefore, CO_2 levels were found to be significantly higher than those associated with comfort ($\leqslant 1000$ ppm), and averaged 1565 and 1756 ppm on smoking and nonsmoking flights respectively. Other studies have confirmed this trend.

As well as being a source of annoyance, tobacco smoke has been cited as the cause of inflight headaches, eye, nose and throat irritation, and breathing problems. In a recent discussion paper, however, it was argued that coexisting factors such as low relative humidity, high ozone levels and even hypoxia could equally well be to blame, and that evidence to the contrary was not available.[12] Of more serious concern is the well publicised belief that exposure to tobacco smoke increases the risk of lung cancer.[13] Many ground based studies, as well as the Geomet study,[11] have attempted to quantify this risk, but the available data, even though much is very poorly analysed and based on faulty assumptions, have not so far supported a relationship between environmental tobacco smoke (ETS) and chronic ill health of any kind. It has been said that "With regard to the health effects hypothesized for ETS, scientific data are quantitatively and qualitatively inadequate to estimate hazard and, equally importantly, to justify prohibition of smoking in airliners".[12] Nevertheless, it is reasonable to conclude that tobacco smoke and other cabin pollutants do not represent a great threat to health, and that their effects are in any case confounded by other factors. Furthermore, although increased ventilation and filtration may improve matters, the volume and flow of circulating air is already high; and passenger segregation appears to be reasonably effective. A total ban on smoking on *all* aircraft would instantly improve matters subjectively; such measures are being actively considered. For example, the congressional ban on smoking in the United States now affects 92% of all flights by American carriers, including international routes,[11] and in 1993 British Airways began a nosmoking trial on one of its services to Hong Kong.

Finally, although not directly related to the quality of cabin air, the potentially harmful effects of ultraviolet radiation on the skin of flight deck crew members has been of concern. Inflight measurements have shown that during flights of several hours' duration (in Boeing 737 and 767 aircraft) the amount of ultraviolet radiation recorded in the cockpit was no more than that received during 1–2 min in the outside air at sea level. Consequently, it was concluded that the risk of developing skin cancer from this cause is no greater for flight deck crew than for anyone else.[14]

Control of disease

The speed and convenience of modern air travel, and the vast numbers of people using the facility, make prevention of intercontinental transmission of disease a major undertaking. There is little doubt that air travel has made a tremendous impact on disease patterns throughout the world: in the United Kingdom, the continued increase in the yearly incidence of malaria is just one example.[15] The purpose of the WHO international health regulations, to which most countries are bound without reservation, is "to ensure the maximum security against the international spread of disease with a minimum interference with world traffic."[16] To this end, articles of the regulations apply to all aircraft and to their ports of entry and exit. The regulations outline the routine preventive and organisational measures to be adopted and describe the wide ranging epidemiological reporting system that allows appropriate steps to be instituted promptly to control any outbreak of disease. The quarantinable diseases of plague, cholera, and yellow fever, and the control of malaria, are governed specifically by the international health regulations, but more generally the regulations require that acceptable standards of preventive medicine and hygiene are met. (Regulations governing smallpox were also included until 1981 when the WHO declared the world to be free of the disease.) Thus the health administration of each country must ensure that airports have supplies of pure water and wholesome food for consumption both on the premises and on board aircraft, together with effective sanitation arrangements.

Airports must be free of rodents and mosquitoes, and wherever possible sufficient medical and supporting staff should be employed to implement all the regulations. Some airports in each country (the number depends on the volume of international traffic) are designated as "sanitary airports" where, in addition to the usual requirements, there must be an organised medical service with facilities for the transport, isolation, and care of known or suspected infected passengers. Facilities for disinsecting, disinfection, and other necessary procedures must be available, as must the facility within the airport or nearby to vaccinate against cholera and yellow fever. There must also be a bacteriological laboratory on site or within easy access. Sanitary airports, even when located in endemic areas, are regarded as infection free for the purpose of international travel. Finally, the health administration must designate some airports as having direct transit areas, under the control of health personnel, where passengers en route may be segregated.

Further articles of the international health regulations govern health measures to be adopted on departure, en route, and on arrival. It is generally regarded as axiomatic that no person suffering, or suspected of suffering, from any infectious disease may travel on commercial airlines, and this is a requirement of the regulations. The justification for, and logic behind, this all embracing view has been challenged by a medical representative of Air France on the grounds that mistakes or arbitrary judgements may be made and that only a small proportion of infected passengers are known to the airline before travel: the risk of spread of disease from the large, unknown reservoir of infected people remains.[17] Instead, reliance on normal airline health measures is recommended, and it is suggested that only those passengers suffering from diseases characterised by vomiting or diarrhoea should be refused passage. Nevertheless, the regulations state the need to prevent embarkation of agents of infection or disease vectors on passengers, in baggage, and on aircraft themselves, and most airlines comply with this.

Occupants of an aircraft in transit through a country, if disembarked en route, and waiting in a direct transit area, cannot be

123

subjected to any health measure apart from a medical examination. Nothing capable of causing an epidemic disease must be allowed to fall from an aircraft while in flight. On arrival, "free pratique" (that is, permission for an aircraft to disembark passengers and commence unloading/loading) must be given unless there is good reason to suspect that a disease may be introduced or spread. An arriving aircraft and its occupants may, however, be subject to medical examination and any appropriate health measures enforced.

Health conditions on board an arriving aircraft are documented by the pilot, or an authorised deputy, in the health part of the General Aircraft Declaration, which must be surrendered to the airport health authority.

Pest control

Other regulations lay down the procedures for destroying pests on board aircraft. *Disinsecting* covers measures taken to kill insect vectors of human disease. These measures must be applied to any aircraft leaving an endemic malarial area, other mosquito borne disease area, or an area where insecticide resistant mosquitoes are present, or to one leaving an infected area en route to an area in which the vector species has been eradicated. The standard of materials (usually synthetic pyrethroid aerosols) to be used is laid down in an annex to the international health regulations and must be harmless to humans and to aircraft structures. They must also be efficient and, as with all other health procedures relating to international travel, cause minimum disruption to aircraft occupants and flight operations. Disinsecting may be carried out well before departure or on arrival, but both of these methods have disadvantages. For example, spraying after arrival is uncomfortable for passengers who may have already been exposed to a live vector during the flight. The method preferred by the WHO is to spray the aircraft cabin, external bays, wheels, and freight areas at the last airport before landing in the country which requires the procedure. Single use aerosols are discharged by the crew as near the time of departure as possible—the so called "blocks away" method. Many health authorities insist on the production of the discharged aerosols on arrival as proof of use. The importance of external treatment was graphically demonstrated a few years ago when 84% of the mosquitoes, 93% of the flies, and 99% of the beetles placed in plastic cages in the wheel arches of a Boeing 747 survived flights at altitudes of 12 042 m (39 500 ft), where the outside air temperature was −54°C.[18]

Disinfestation is the term used to describe the methods adopted to deal with other pests. Fumigation at regular (6-weekly) intervals keeps cockroaches, the most common pest of all, in check and is recommended whether or not they have been seen. Rodents, which are quite capable of eating aircraft wiring and other structures, must be destroyed by full fumigation when their presence is suspected. Methyl bromide is commonly used and effective but its use is time consuming and requires very strict safety precautions; authorised contractors must provide a certificate of clearance before re-entry to the aircraft is allowed. Disinfection and deratting procedures will be required on arrival if a person suffering from plague has been on board.

Aircrew scheduling

The need to operate commercial airlines worldwide for 24 hours each day inevitably leads to problems of aircrew management: to the stresses of flying an aircraft must be added those of unsocial and irregular hours, time zone (transmeridian), climatic and cultural changes, sleep disturbances, and alterations to circadian rhythms. Fatigue is the main danger, because a decline in performance is likely to accompany it. The economic and operational requirements of an airline must be balanced against these undesirable factors, but good aircrew scheduling is essential to the health, morale, and safety of aircrew: the narrow area wherein lies safe and economic management has concerned the civil aviation industry for many years.

In 1973 the Bader committee on flight time limitations,[19] while not attributing any aircraft accident in the United Kingdom to fatigue, nevertheless recommended considerable constraints on aircrew scheduling. These constraints, which were updated, clarified, and simplified in 1982,[20] are applied statutorily by the Civil Aviation Authority and include limitations on the maximum flying duty period, minimum rest periods, maximum scheduled duty hours, and minimum cumulative off duty periods. Before this revision, the United Kingdom's proposed flight schedules had to be submitted by the airline management to the Flight Times Limitation Board before introduction. But, as practices became well established and the need for routine guidance declined, the part played by the Board diminished until, in 1987, it was disbanded. The advisory role on flight time limitations previously filled by the Board is now undertaken by the Operations Advisory Committee, which has been the source of advice to the Civil Aviation Authority on all operational matters since 1985. Other countries have similar limitations, and within such frameworks airlines operate schedules which are further restricted by the need to please passengers and to comply with night flying bans, peak hour saturation, and political influences on route planning. In addition, flight time limitations usually reflect conditions acceptable to industrial bodies rather than to medical advisers. The commercial need to keep aircraft flying, and so earning revenue, and the requirements of engineering schedules for airframe and engine inspections and checks are also relevant considerations.

Transmeridian travel

Notwithstanding the commercial bias of present scheduling practice, disturbances of sleep and the problems of transmeridian travel are of particular concern to aviation medicine specialists. Adequate sleep is necessary for aircrew to adapt to irregular work, while alterations in circadian rhythms may reduce effectiveness and impair performance.

Aircrew operating long haul schedules alter their sleep patterns to cope with irregular hours and time zone changes by adopting a mixture of short naps and intermediate and long periods of sleep.[21] Although there may be some reduction in total sleep time, this pattern appears to be acceptable and, based upon the favourable performance results of a NASA study into rotating sleep periods of 40 min while cruising at altitude, the Federal Aviation Administration is even considering whether to allow airlines to institute structured napping.[22] Should a cumulative loss of sleep accompany the disturbed sleep pattern, however, the implications for psychomotor, and hence operational, performance are more serious.[23-25]

Aircrew are just as susceptible to the problems of re-entrainment of their circadian rhythms after transmeridian travel, and are as prone to the problems of jet lag as their passengers (see chapter 3). But for aircrew the important changes are those associated with performance levels.

Many mental skills, including vigilance, choice reaction time, and simulator performance, rise to a peak during the day between 1200 and 2100 and then fall to a minimum between 0300 and 0600.

Results of memory tests peak in the morning and then fall steadily.[26] Increased levels of arousal, as a result of flying stress, may partly compensate for decreased performance during troughs in the rhythms and during prolonged periods of work, but if circadian rhythmicity is disrupted by time zone changes then even the usually sound advice to avoid potentially hazardous manoeuvres, such as night takeoff and landing, may not prevent reduced flying efficiency and thus flight safety. The rest time required for resynchronisation may be calculated from a knowledge of flight duration and direction, times of departure and arrival, and the number of time zones crossed,[27] but aircrew schedules so derived are often commercially impossible to achieve in practice. In the absence of ideal solutions aircrew are recommended to keep sleep deficit to a minimum by using any opportunity to take naps.[26] Remaining on home base time is also suggested, as is a return home as soon as possible, but such advice is difficult to follow unless the airline scheduling department is aware of these problems and can roster crews to allow them to progress as quickly as possible.

Disturbances in sleep patterns are also a feature of short haul schedules because the times of commuter flights are planned to accommodate travellers and their normal office hours. Adaptation to the encroachment of schedules on early morning or late evening sleep is achieved by varying the length of sleep at each end of the duty period. Short naps are not a feature of this adaptation and total sleep, over months, for these aircrew is similar to that for non shift workers.[21] Nevertheless, shorter and poorer sleep periods are a feature of short haul operations, along with recognisable mood changes.[28]

Cabin crew

While most investigative work in this area has concentrated on the effects on flight deck crew, it must be remembered that cabin staff have a physically demanding job and are subject to similar temporal and environmental stresses. These are becoming increasingly relevant as aircraft capable of flying continuously for longer periods of time than ever before come into service. Furthermore, it has been demonstrated that correctly trained cabin staff can improve such vital activities as aircraft evacuation by 50%,[28] so adequate attention to their training needs and to the scheduling of workloads is essential. A plea has also been made for increased assertiveness on the part of cabin staff because there is evidence that intervention by knowledgeable cabin staff could have averted several aircraft accidents in the recent past: an inflight emergency is no time for reticence.[29] Thus, words written over 12 years ago, when cabin attendants were "universally recognized ... as the primary cabin safety factor in the event of in-flight or ground emergencies"[30] have even more relevance today.

Emergency considerations

Oxygen

The oxygen requirements for civil aircraft, both those which are capable of being pressurised and those which fly unpressurised, are laid down in the Air Navigation Order.[31] For example, pressurised aircraft that fly above 7620 m (25 000 ft) must carry enough oxygen for continuous use by the flight deck crew for at least 2 hours in the event of a decompression to cabin altitudes above 3048 m (10 000 ft), as well as an emergency supply for cabin attendants and all passengers for at least 10 min whenever the cabin altitude exceeds 3658 m (12 000 ft). A separate therapeutic supply, adequate for at least two passengers at any one time, must also be available. Most airlines comfortably exceed these requirements to avoid problems during testing, due to leakage, and with overseas supply.

Fire

The ideal solution to aircraft fires is to prevent them occurring or, if this is not possible, to extinguish them immediately at source. The use of modern kerosene fuels and fire resistant hydraulic fluids has helped to reduce the likelihood of ignition, while automatic extinguishers in the engines and fuel cutoff valves help to prevent spread. Despite such improvements, fire, fumes and smoke in the cabins of aircraft which have successfully crash landed or aborted takeoff continue to claim lives. Toxic fumes, particularly hydrogen cyanide and carbon monoxide, resulting from pyrolysis of cabin furnishings[32] are the greatest single threat to the safety of passengers and crew in an aircraft that has landed successfully with a fire on board. Such fumes, along with heat and smoke, incapacitate potential survivors and probably cause death within 2–5 min.[33]

Although excellent, almost fireproof materials have been available for some time, and wide ranging recommendations encourage their use in cabin furniture, expense was often given as the reason for not incorporating them. A series of fatal accidents in the early 1980s, involving fire on board aircraft after successful landings or aborted takeoffs, as in the British Airtours Boeing 737 disaster at Manchester in 1985, stimulated the aviation authorities into *requiring* improved safety features. Regulations now require the installation of seats incorporating materials that both resist and block fire, smoke detectors and automatic fire extinguishers in toilets, as well as the general use of less toxic materials in cabin furnishings. In the United Kingdom, the Air Navigation Order has been amended to require, from 1 January 1990, the provision of protective breathing equipment (smokehoods) for flight deck crew and cabin staff. Such equipment is to provide protection for at least 15 min. The provision of smoke hoods or masks for *all* was just one of Hill's recommendations for improvement following his analysis of factors which impeded successful escape from the British Airtours crash. The others were upper torso restraint, floor level lighting, no seats in exit paths, wider passageways, and fuller passenger briefings (to include, for example, counting the number of seat rows to the nearest exit, and explicit instructions for those seated next to exits).[33] The regulating authorities had at least some of these measures in hand already, and others are under discussion.

In 1991, the Civil Aviation Authority rejected the use of smokehoods for passenger use, claiming that they would kill more than they saved.[34] The drawbacks identified by the authority mainly revolve around the time likely to be taken by a crash victim to don a potentially complex piece of equipment, however good its design and however thorough the briefing on it may be.[35] In addition, the ability of smokehoods to protect physiologically as well as toxicologically is vital and must be assured. It is clearly beyond dispute that "some aircraft fires are survivable but that people have died and been injured because they could not escape in time",[36] so greater efforts must be made to seek a satisfactory solution. Finally, the decision to provide smokehoods for all occupants of all aircraft will be influenced by other constraints, not least of which will be cost, weight and bulk.

Other improvements are also being assessed. For example, and most importantly, a research programme into water deluge systems was recently agreed by the Federal Aviation Administration, the Civil Aviation Authority, Transport Canada, and the European Joint Airworthiness Authority; such systems have now been refined to the point where they can be considered realistically. A ruling may be possible in 1993, which would allow regulations to be in place by 1994/95.[37] The size of the spray droplets is crucial: droplets must be small enough to extract heat, yet of a size which is not instantly vaporised. Large droplets not only mean weight crippling penalties, but also encourage spread of fire. British Petroleum's solution, for example, relies on careful production of a mist of water droplets with mean diameters of 80–200 μm. Trials of this fire spray technology have demonstrated that sprays deployed from the top and sides of a cabin can significantly delay first the combustion of cabin furnishings and then the spread of fire. Temperature is reduced, as is the level of water soluble toxic material (by 80%). The system is so efficient that just 100 l of water could protect an aircraft with 120 seats.[38]

Impact

Incapacitation can also occur as a result of injury from flying debris, as was the case in the British Midland Boeing 737 disaster on the M1 motorway in January 1989. In this accident 47 people died and 79 survived. Many of the fatalities were caused by massive multisystem trauma at points where the aircraft fractured, but the severe posterior head injuries seen in many of the dead (24) and in some of the survivors (18) were caused by impacts from the overhead bins, all but one of which broke loose. In all, 42 of the 118 passengers had posterior head trauma. It was concluded that many of these injuries would not have occurred if aircraft materials and structural design had advanced rather more over the past 30 years.[39] As has been the case so often in the past, the official report on this accident called for a re-evaluation of floor and cabin furniture design, and of alternative seating and harness configurations.[40] In this instance, however, rearward facing seats would merely have resulted in anterior rather than posterior injuries. But it is of great relevance that those passengers who adopted a fully braced precrash posture were significantly less likely to have suffered head injury or to have been concussed.[41] Demonstration and practice of the brace position during pretakeoff briefings should be introduced; particularly because it would be a relatively easy addition to the now customary delivery by video. Other improvements in this area would be more difficult to achieve, both practically and in terms of cost–benefit. It can only be a matter of time before seats and cabin floors are strengthened, restraints improved, and overhead lockers eliminated or strengthened.[42] It would also be of help if their contents did not include heavy but mobile glass bottles of duty free drink.

Emergency escape

In the United Kingdom the Civil Aviation Authority requires that escape from a burning aircraft should be accomplished within 90 s. This standard was derived from simulated escapes from aircraft that were not on fire, that were not filled with smoke, and in which at least half the exits were available and working correctly. The time limit is helped somewhat by emergency lighting, large doors, and double aisles in wide bodied jets, but the requirement is clearly taxing. Furthermore, having reached an exit from which an automatic slide has been deployed successfully, the occupants are still at risk of collision and injury[43]—a risk that is clearly increased if the slide fails to deploy, deploys incorrectly, is destroyed, or if survivors are not quickly led away from the foot of the slide.

Until recently, the Federal Aviation Administration also required these specifications to be met, but has now *reduced* the time to evacuate a stricken aircraft from 90 to just 62 s![44] Reassuringly, under the new procedures, a 405-passenger aircraft was recently evacuated in 56 s. In parallel with this modification, however, is another which requires tests of escape slides to be carried out independently of cabin evacuation trials; a move which followed an evacuation assessment by McDonnell Douglas in October 1991 during which one woman fractured her neck and was paralysed, and a further 46 people were injured!

Conclusion

This chapter summarises some of the areas in which the airline/airport doctor might be concerned. The clinical and occupational health and safety of aircrew and passengers are of obvious importance, but it must be remembered that airlines and airports require an enormous ground based supporting staff. This "keep them flying brigade" has been estimated to comprise about 70% of airline employees, and to require vast occupational medicine support; not the least part of which is the ever-increasing burden

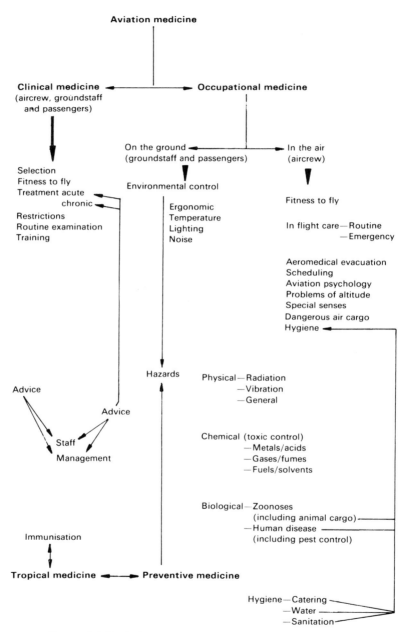

FIG 9.1—Scope of civil aviation medicine.

of regulating laws and requirements.[45] The doctor who chooses to work in this specialty must provide a comprehensive service for this population. In addition, other medical aspects must be considered in cargo operations, including those of dangerous air cargo and, in conjunction with veterinary colleagues, the carriage of animals. Figure 9·1 shows the scope of the civil aviation medicine specialist.

1 Anonymous. *Occupational health and safety in civil aviation*. Geneva: International Labour Office, 1977: 5.
2 Learmont D. Is nothing safe? *Flight International* 1991; **141**: (29 Jan.) 20–6.
3 Preston FS. An outbreak of gastroenteritis in aircrew. *Aviat Space Environ Med* 1968; **39**: 519–21.
4 Peffers ASR, Food sanitation and air safety. *Aviat Space Environ Med* 1976; **46**: 1107–8.
5 Bailey J. *Guide to hygiene and sanitation in aviation*. Geneva: World Health Organization, 1977.
6 *The food safety act 1990*. London: HMSO, 1990.
7 WHO. *International standards for drinking water*, 3rd edn. Geneva: World Health Organization, 1971.
8 Rondle CJM, Ramesh B, Krahn JB, Sherriff R. Cholera: possible infection from aircraft effluent. *J Hyg (Camb)* 1978; **81**: 361–71.
9 Minerva. Views. *BMJ* 1988; **296**: 362.
10 Smith A. Smoke free flying (editorial). *BMJ* 1988; **297**: 1001.
11 Geomet Technologies Inc. *Airliner cabin environment: contaminant measurements, health risks and mitigation options*. Washington: US Department of Transportation, 1989.
12 Crawford WA, Holcomb LC. Environmental tobacco smoke (ETS) in airliners—a health hazard evaluation. *Aviat Space Environ Med*. 1991; **62**: 580–6.
13 US Surgeon General. *The health consequences of involuntary smoking*. Rockville, MD: US Department of Health and Human Services, 1986.
14 Diffey BL, Roscoe AH. Exposure to solar ultraviolet radiation in flight. *Aviat Space Environ Med* 1990; **61**: 1032–5.
15 Bradley DJ, Warhurst DC, Blaze M, Smith V. Malaria imported into the UK 1989 and 1990. *Communicable disease report* 1991; **1**: R45–8.
16 WHO. *International health regulations (1969)*, 2nd annotated edn. Geneva: World Health Organization, 1974.
17 Perin M. Transportation in commercial aircraft of passengers having contagious diseases. *Aviat Space Environ Med* 1976; **47**: 1109–13.
18 *Bull World Health Organ* 1987; **65**: 659–62.
19 Bader D. *Report of the committee on flight time limitations*. London: Civil Aviation Authority, 1973.
20 Civil Aviation Authority: *The avoidance of excessive fatigue in aircrews—guide to requirements*, 2nd edn. London: Civil Aviation Authority, 1982. (CAP 371.)
21 Nicholson AN, Stone BM. *Sleep and wakefulness handbook for flight medical officers*, 2nd edn. Neuilly-sur-Seine, France: NATO Advisory Group for Aerospace Research and Development, 1987. (AGARDograph No 270.)
22 Barnett R. Nap time for pilots. *Travel and Leisure* 1993; **March:** 202.
23 Fiorica V, Higgins EA, Iampietro PF, Lategola MT, Davis AW. Physiological responses of men during sleep deprivation. *J Appl Physiol* 1968; **24**: 167–76.
24 Spencer MB, Stone BM, Rogers AS, Nicholson AN. Circadian rhythmicity and sleep of aircrew during polar schedules. *Aviat Space Environ Med* 1991; **62**: 3–13.
25 Samel A, Wegmann HM, Summa W, Naumann M. Sleep patterns in aircrew operating on the polar route between Germany and East Asia. *Aviat Space Environ Med* 1991; **62**: 661–9.
26 Klein KE, Wegmann HM. *Significance of circadian rhythms in aerospace operations*. Neuilly-sur-Seine, France: NATO Advisory Group for Aerospace Research and Development, 1980. (AGARDograph No 247.)
27 Mohler SR. Physiological index as an aid in developing airline pilot scheduling patterns. *Aviat Space Environ Med* 1976; **47**: 238–47.

28 Chidchester TR. Trends and individual differences in response to short-haul flight operations. *Aviat Space Environ Med* 1990; **61**: 132–8.

29 Anonymous. One crew or two. *Flight International* 1993; **143** (Number 4357): 3,9.

30 Alter JD, Mohler SR. Preventive medicine aspects and health promotion programs for flight attendants. *Aviat Space Environ Med* 1980; **51**: 168–75.

31 Statutory Instruments 1987, No 2062. Civil Aviation. The Air Navigation (Second Amendment) Order 1987: 6–8 (Scale K2).

32 Mohler SR. Air crash survival: injuries and evacuation toxic hazards. *Aviat Space Environ Med* 1975; **46**: 86–8.

33 Hill IR. An analysis of factors impeding passenger escape from aircraft fires. *Aviat Space Environ Med* 1990; **61**: 261–5.

34 Civil Aviation Authority. *Improving passenger survivability in aircraft fires: a review.* London: Civil Aviation Authority, 1991. (CAP 586.)

35 Edgington K. Making air crashes more survivable (letter). *BMJ* 1992; **305**: 119.

36 Hill IR. Smoke hoods in aeroplanes (editorial). *BMJ* 1992; **304**: 1326.

37 Elliott S. Water mist decision due in May. *Flight International* 1993; **143** (Number 4354): 10.

38 Baldwin B. The water safety curtain. *Aerospace* 1993; **20**: 18–19.

39 White BD, Firth JL, Rowles JM, NLDB Study Group. The effects of structural failure on injuries sustained in the M1 Boeing 737 disaster, January 1989. *Aviat Space Environ Med* 1993; **64**: 95–102.

40 The Department of Transport. Air Accidents Investigation Branch. *Report on the accident to Boeing 737-400 G-OBME near Kegworth, Leicestershire on 8 January 1989.* Farnborough: Royal Aircraft Establishment 1990. Aircraft Accident Report 4/90.

41 White BD, Firth JL, Rowles JM, NLDB Study Group. The effects of brace position on injuries sustained in the M1 Boeing 737 disaster, January 1989. *Aviat Space Environ Med* 1993; **64**: 103–9.

42 Gloag D. Making air crashes more survivable (editorial). *BMJ* 1992; **304**: 1325–6.

43 Pollard DW. Injuries in air transport emergency evacuations. *Aviat Space Environ Med* 1979; **50**: 943–7.

44 Anonymous. FAA modifies its rules for evacuation test. *Flight International*. 1993; **143** (Number 4354): 13.

45 DeHart RL. Occupational medicine support for international air carriers. *Aviat Space Environ Med* 1990; **61**: 67–70.

10
Is the crew fit to fly?

Look to your health; and if you have it, praise God, and value it next to a good conscience, for health is the second blessing that we mortals are capable of; a blessing that money cannot buy.

Izaak Walton (1593–1683)

For those who earn their livelihood by flying, medical fitness is of prime importance because safety in flight and future financial security will both be adversely affected by ill health. Redundancy apart, medical disqualification is the most frequent reason for the premature involuntary termination of an airline pilot's career and, contrary to popular belief, few airlines are able to offer alternative ground employment to those so affected. In the United Kingdom alone between 20 and 30 professional pilots' licences are lost each year for medical reasons, usually because there is an unacceptable risk that the holder may become incapacitated while in control of an aircraft. This figure translates into 2–2·5 denials of licence per 1000 professional aircrew in the United Kingdom, and compares with losses of about 4 per 1000 in the United States, France and Japan. The lower rate is a reflection of the waiver policy the Civil Aviation Authority has, and its progressive attitude towards disposition of cardiovascular problems.

Inflight incapacitation

Incapacitation may be sudden or insidious. Sudden incapacitation may be obvious to other crew members but may result in complete loss of function and be extremely dangerous if it occurs during a critical phase of takeoff or landing. Insidious incapacitation may not be obvious to those afflicted or, more importantly, to other crew members. Both may jeopardise the safe operation of the aircraft, but data on incidence—particularly of sudden incapacitation—are scarce, although several studies give further insight to the extent of the problem.

135

The incidence of insidious incapacitation is difficult to assess but it is reported to be more common than sudden incapacitation.[1] Fortunately, the occurrence is usually transient and is statistically more likely to occur during a relatively safe phase of flight. Gastrointestinal disturbance is the most common cause of such incapacitation,[2] but the causes of subtle or partial loss of cerebral function are more dangerous and may include reactive hypoglycaemia and psychological factors.[1] In 1991, the results of a survey conducted by the International Federation of Airline Pilots Associations were published.[3] Of 4345 pilots from 97 airlines in 16 countries, 1251 (29%) had experienced at least one incident of incapacitation while operating an aircraft, which required someone else to take control: statistics which were remarkably similar to those in a survey conducted in 1967.[2] Almost one-half the pilots thought that safety had been affected to some degree. Gastrointestinal disturbances were once again the most common cause (58%), followed by nasal and sinus congestion, headaches, faintness or general weakness.

In 1990, Air France reported the results of a 20 year survey of sudden inflight incapacitation affecting pilots and engineers.[4] During this period, 10 cases occurred in a total of 1800 cockpit crew each flying an average of 600 hours per year: epilepsy (2), cardiac problems (2), duodenal haemorrhage (2), and one case each of viral labyrinthitis, hypoglycaemia, carbon dioxide poisoning and hypoxia. A survey 6 years earlier of 36 000 pilots at risk had revealed 26 major incidents but no associated accidents over a 10 year period.[5] In this series there were 10 cases of myocardial ischaemia, seven of epileptiform fits, six of syncope, and three of cerebral haemorrhage. In the world of general aviation, sudden inflight incapacitation has been estimated to cause three accidents per 1000 overall, and 15 of every 1000 fatal accidents.[6]

These authors (and others) agree that the most effective way to reduce the potentially lethal risks of these events depends particularly on the ability of all aircrew to recognise problems in their colleagues, and to take appropriate remedial action. Appreciation of this need led to the introduction of incapacitation training in the United Kingdom (mandatory since 1973) and elsewhere, and has been demonstrably successful: for example, although incapacitation still occurs, there has been no scheduled multicrew aircraft accident attributable to cardiovascular incapacitation for 20 years (about 250 million flying hours).[7] The relative infrequency of serious incidents of any kind must also be the result, at least in part, of the strict medical selection of aircrew and of subsequent regular and rigorous medical evaluations.

Regulation of aviation safety and aircrew licensing

The regulation of aviation safety throughout the world is the responsibility of a United Nations agency, the International Civil Aviation Organization. This body issues international standards and recommended practices which cover all aspects of airline safety, and which all nations are bound by treaty to uphold. These standards and recommended practices including those governing personnel licensing, are usually general statements which are then amplified and embodied in national regulations and administered by individual national agencies. In the United Kingdom, this responsibility rests with the Civil Aviation Authority, while the Federal Aviation Administration is the corresponding agency in the United States. Any nation is free to enhance these standards (and indeed individual airlines can also increase licensing requirements on commercial grounds) but any deviation or reduction has to be notified to the International Civil Aviation Organization.

The European office of the Organization is located in Paris, and is one of seven regional offices worldwide. In support of harmonisation of European aviation standards, the Organization has established a European Civil Aviation Conference, which has in turn appointed committees to produce the new regulations. One of these, the Flight Crew Licensing Committee, has specialist medical subcommittees reporting to it. Eventually, the deliberations of the European Conference and its committees will, among other things, lead to the promulgation of new medical licensing standards for Europe under the auspices of the European Joint Aviation Authority, although individual national agencies will retain full executive and administrative responsibilities. Comprehensive guidance on the new standards, which are to be more detailed than those of the International Civil Aviation Organization, will be given in the *European manual of civil aviation medicine* intended to replace the former's manual: the extant source of guidance.[8]

Perhaps not surprisingly, the draft medical standards (some of which call for additional and costly testing of debatable clinical or safety value for licensing purposes (for example haemoglobin estimation at every examination, and 5-yearly blood lipid analysis), while others call for more intensive specialised examinations of, for example, the eyes and ears) have attracted considerable criticism within the United Kingdom from the airlines, and from professional organisations such as the British Airline Pilots Association. Two more ad hoc Flight Crew Licensing subcommittees have been formed to help deal with this reaction, but the original intent to have the Joint Aviation Authority regulations in place by January 1996 now looks hopelessly optimistic. It is likely that introduction will be delayed by at least 1 year and probably longer.[9] Thus, for the time being, the Civil Aviation Authority will continue both to oversee initial and periodic medical examination of aircrew, and to be responsible through its medical department for the maintenance of medical standards. It should be noted that in its industrial response to the harmonisation proposals, the United Kingdom stands alone: the other 11 nations involved (many of which already have increased requirements of the kind proposed) have agreed them—including the many liberal approaches carried through by the Civil Aviation Authority.

Initial examination

Aircrew are examined by doctors who are usually general practitioners and are often private pilots themselves, and who have undergone postgraduate training in aviation medicine. Under the Joint Aviation Authority harmonisation proposals such training will be carried out at designated aeromedical centres, and will involve up to 50 hours of teaching. In the United Kingdom, courses for the certificate and diploma in aviation medicine, which in large part already meet the requirements, are conducted at the Royal Air Force Institute of Aviation Medicine, and holders of either qualification are eligible for appointment as an authorised medical examiner (AME). Once appointed, an authorised medical examiner holding the certificate in aviation medicine can examine private pilots, while diplomates can also examine professional aircrew. A register of examiners is maintained by the Civil Aviation Authority, and there is usually a waiting list. The examiners issue three classes of medical certificate (table 10.1), valid for periods of 6–60 months (table 10.2) depending on the type of licence held and the applicant's age. As noted above, basic minimum medical standards are laid down by the International Civil

TABLE 10.1—Classes of medical certificate issued by the Civil Aviation Authority

Class	Licence	
1	Airline transport pilot Commercial pilot Air traffic control officer Flight engineer Flight navigator (rarely taken up)	Also eligible for licences as student and private pilots
2	Basic commercial pilot* Commercial pilot (balloon) Private pilot (flight instruction)	
3	Private pilot Student pilot Motor glider pilot	

*Holders of a basic commercial pilot licence are allowed to undertake employment other than for public transport (such as aerial work, crop spraying, banner towing, display flying, and flight instruction).

Aviation Organization, but each member country is free to impose higher standards for its own national licences.

The initial examination of professional aircrew and air traffic control officers (that is, classes 1 and 2) is carried out at the Civil Aviation Authority's own medical centre. At other examinations the applicant must meet certain medical criteria that are defined by the authority's medical department in a handbook provided for use by its authorised medical examiners. The standards for class 1 certificates are higher overall than for classes 2 and 3. When the fitness of a private pilot is in doubt, an authorised examiner may seek local consultant opinion to help decide whether a medical certificate can be issued. Professional aircrew and air traffic control officers who fail to meet the standards at subsequent periodic examination must be referred to the authority for further assessment.

Although not part of the medical licensing requirements, it is of interest to note that, from January 1991, all applicants for a pilot's licence (from private pilot to airline transport pilot) have also to pass a written examination in human performance and limitations, which covers topics in aviation physiology and psychology.

Visual function

The need for high visual standards is obvious, and ophthalmic

139

TABLE 10.2—Current requirements for medical certification and recertification

Licence	Age (years)	Duration of validity of medical certificate	Electrocardiogram*		Audiogram		Visual acuity	Chest radiograph	Physical, visual, and auditory standards
			Age (years)	Renewal interval	Age (years)	Renewal interval			
Airline transport pilot	All	6 months	<30	5 years			At least 6/9 in each eye, with maximum correction, if needed, of ±3·00 dioptres ese		As on initial examination
Commercial pilot	>40	6 months	30–39	2 years					
Commercial pilot	<40	1 year	40–49	1 year	<40	5 years			
			>50	6 months					
Air traffic control officer	All	1 year	<30	5 years			Uncorrected vision at least 6/60	Initial only, unless clinically indicated	
Flight engineer		1 year	30–39	2 years	>40	3 years			
Flight navigator		1 year	>40	1 year					
Basic commercial pilot			<40	IO			At least 6/9 in each eye, with maximum correction, if needed, of ±5·00 dioptres ese		
Basic commercial pilot	<40	2 years	40–49	2 years	Not required unless clinically indicated				
Basic commercial pilot	40–59	1 year	50–59	1 year					
Commercial pilot (balloons)	>60	6 months	>60	6 months					
Private pilot (instructor)									
Student/private pilot	<40	5 years	<40	NR	Not required unless clinically indicated, except on initial issue of private pilot's licence instrument rating		At least 6/12 in each eye, with maximum correction, if needed, of ±5·00 dioptres ese. Myopia of up to −8·00 dioptres may be waived	Not required unless clinically indicated	
Student/private pilot	40–49	2 years	At first PME after age 40 then 40–49	4 years					
Student/private pilot	50–69	1 year	50–59	2 years					
Student/private pilot	>70	6 months	60–69	1 year					
Glider instructor			>70	6 months					

*Required at initial examination for class 1 and 2 licences
PME = Periodic medical examination
IO = Initial only, unless clinically indicated

problems are a common cause of rejection in applicants for ab initio commercial pilot training. Safe colour vision is essential and must be verified at the initial examination for all medical classes by Ishihara plates. Candidates who fail this test should be referred to a specialist for a lantern test because they may still possess sufficient colour discrimination to operate an aircraft safely. Standards of visual acuity are laid down according to the type of licence to be issued, and these permit spectacles to be worn provided that the vision is correctable to the level of acuity defined in the visual standard (see table 10.2). Contact lenses are accepted provided that all day non-flying tolerance has been established for at least 3 months. Spare spectacles must also be carried by all those who have visual correction aids whether contact lenses or ordinary spectacles. Evidence is also required that other visual variables are within normal limits.

Cardiovascular function

Although many cardiovascular abnormalities may come to light at an initial medical examination, where they are often not compatible with the issue of a licence (particularly in the case of middle aged private pilots), their diagnosis at periodic examination gives rise to considerable problems of disposal. Accordingly, these conditions are discussed below. Two areas of cardiovascular function are, however, of particular interest at the initial examination: the electrocardiogram, and the question of hypertension.

A resting electrocardiogram is required at initial examination for class 1 and 2 licences but only for a class 3 licence if the applicant is aged 40 or over. (The subsequent periodicity of electrocardiographic examinations depends on age and class of licence: see table 10.2.) The electrocardiograms must then be scrutinised by a cardiologist or physician experienced in their interpretation; and those of professional aircrew are read centrally by Civil Aviation Authority cardiologists with access to previous records.

In the United States, in a move designed to reduce this physician-intensive and somewhat onerous task, the Federal Aviation Administration instigated central and automated reading of electrocardiograms from all class 1 licence examinations from August 1987. American authorised medical examiners are required to transmit electrocardiograms electronically to the Civil Aeromedical Institute where they are "screened" by computer: abnormal traces are reread manually, as are the 2% of traces which fail

141

because of technical errors. By March 1990, the Institute had nearly 138 000 records on file, and the scheme has greatly reduced the Administration's staffing and paperwork costs: the cost to the examinee has, however, risen![10]

A normal tracing does not exclude ischaemic heart disease, which should also be sought actively by history and examination. If the initial resting trace is abnormal then further cardiovascular evaluation by a specialist is indicated (see below). Such investigations should be carried out in consultation with the Civil Aviation Authority to ensure that they are appropriate and to avoid undue delay in providing a decision on an applicant's medical eligibility for flying.

Routine exercise electrocardiographic testing of all applicants with normal as well as abnormal resting tracings is unlikely to be worthwhile: indeed, there is no existing requirement for this, as it has been shown that exercise electrocardiography yields a high proportion of false-positive results with poor specificity and reproducibility. In one study, 771 asymptomatic men aged 35–54 with normal resting tracings were exposed to maximal treadmill or Double Master's tests and as a result, 19 men underwent cardiac catheterization but only four showed coronary artery disease.[11] On the other hand, Bruce[12] has stated that the sensitivity and specificity of exercise electrocardiograms are appreciably improved by repeated testing at yearly intervals. More recently, Broustet et al.,[13] while agreeing that routine testing of asymptomatic subjects is nugatory effort, noted that it is a useful screening test in a number of conditions and where the resting electrocardiogram is equivocal. In these circumstances, a properly performed exercise protocol which reveals little or no change in electrocardiogram at an adequate level of exertion (Stage III of a Bruce treadmill test) is "sufficiently sensitive to exclude the necessity of further investigation".[13] False-positive results can often be clarified by a repeat challenge using glyceryl trinitrate or by exercise scintigraphy without recourse to definitive coronary angiography, although the last is the only way to establish individual risk.

A second area of cardiovascular controversy is in establishing a diagnosis of hypertension (see also below). Although the Civil Aviation Authority provides age related guidelines on acceptable maximum levels of blood pressure, these differ from those of other licensing authorities which has resulted in a confusing variety of standards.[14] Further error on examination is introduced by factors such as anxiety, posture (the authority requires supine blood pressure readings), the use of phase 4 or 5 of the Korotkoff sounds to interpret diastolic pressure (the authority recommends phase 5—that is, cessation of arterial sounds), and other observer errors including digit preference (the tendency for measurements to end in 0 or 5). Controlled hypertension is usually acceptable in the absence of target organ disease provided that treatment is shown to be free from notable side effects in the individual. On-the-job performance testing is often required and other risk factors such as smoking must also be taken into account.

Human immunodeficiency virus

Since its first appearance, infection with human immuno-deficiency virus (HIV) has spread with relentless devastation, so that there are now an estimated 8–10 million people affected worldwide. In the United States alone, approximately 1 million are infected, and there the Centers for Disease Control have predicted that there will be 390 000–480 000 cases of acquired immune deficiency syndrome (AIDS) by the end of 1993. In the United Kingdom the figures are somewhat less alarming, with about 20 000–30 000 infected individuals and a total, at the end of 1992, of just under 7000 cases of AIDS in the 10 years or so since the outbreak began. There is, however, no evidence at present to refute the seemingly inevitable progression from HIV infection to AIDS or AIDS related illness and then to death.

No stratum of human society is unaffected by this pandemic, and it is not surprising that the aviation industry has paid particular attention to the scourge, because the mobility offered by air travel is, in part, responsible. The WHO has declared guidelines for the international traveller (see chapter 3) but these are inappropriate for those doing the transporting.

The concern for aircrew licensing authorities is that part of the early natural history of HIV infection is entry to the central nervous system. In fully established AIDS, neurological destruction is a common finding, but many neuropsychiatric syndromes have also been reported in asymptomatic HIV infected individuals.[15] These syndromes include

● the dementia complex, with cognitive (forgetfulness, confusion, loss of concentration), behavioural (apathy, withdrawal) and

143

motor (impaired visual tracking, balance and tactility) components;

- suicide;
- cerebral infarction;
- neuropathy and myopathy;
- myelopathy and meningitis.

In view of the seriousness of this collection of disorders on the ability of HIV infected aircrew to perform without danger to their passengers and others, and in the complete absence of any neuropsychiatric method of assessing fitness to fly, the Aerospace Medical Association approved the following statement of position in May 1991:

> The Aerospace Medical Association believes the HIV-infected pilot places the flying public at increased and unnecessary risk, and therefore supports testing of pilots for infection by the HIV virus (sic). Individuals confirmed to be so infected should be found medically disqualified for flying duties.[16]

This logic, based on scientific evidence of subtle neuropsychiatric complications of HIV positivity, led the United States navy in September 1987, and air force 1 month later, to adopt a policy of grounding all HIV positive aircrew permanently and without possibility of waiver.[17]

The Aerospace Medical Association statement is not without its critics, and a strong case has been made for the use of sensitive screening tests for early detection of subtle deficits.[18] Concern was also expressed at the apparent conflict between this statement and the stance adopted by the WHO which, in its first consultation on HIV infection, had stated that:

> ... governments, employers and the public can be assured that based on the weight of available scientific evidence, otherwise healthy HIV-1 infected individuals are no more likely to be functionally impaired from a neuropsychiatric viewpoint than uninfected persons.[19]

And in its second consultation, the WHO commented thus:

> Given the evidence ... denial of access to employment ... for otherwise healthy persons solely on the basis of HIV-1 serological status would represent a violation of human rights and lead to broad and destructive social implications.[20]

There is, in fact, no conflict if it is accepted that "otherwise healthy" implies no neuropsychiatric deficit at all: a status that is not possible to establish with tests currently available. Consequently, and mindful of the overriding requirement for "the safe passage of an aircraft", the Aerospace Medical Association's position is probably inevitable until such time as new knowledge dictates otherwise.

The national civil licensing authorities have yet to issue their own definitive guidance on the matter, although the draft Joint Aviation Authority's requirements indicate that while AIDS and AIDS related illnesses will be disqualifying, those who are HIV positive may be recertified subject to frequent review: this is also the position of the Civil Aviation Authority at present. However, many airlines have instituted corporate policies based not only on evidence such as that described above but also on practical and commercial necessity. For example British Airways screens all its aircrew applicants (flight deck and cabin staff), and does not employ any found to be HIV positive on the grounds that staff must be fit for an entire career of worldwide service. Worldwide service, of course, requires immunisation, and department of health guidelines are clear that live vaccine such as that for yellow fever must not be given to the immunologically compromised.[21]

Other conditions

Certain other conditions of importance, including acute or chronic ear disease, unacceptable hearing loss (audiography is required at initial class 1 examinations), and a history of psychiatric disease, must be excluded at initial medical examination. These ailments and others incompatible with the issue of a certificate by an authorised medical examiner are summarised in table 10.3, although the list is not exhaustive.

Other considerations

It is important to appreciate that for commercial reasons the medical standards expected of ab initio recruits by the airlines will usually exceed those defined by the Civil Aviation Authority, which can take into account only the period of validity of the medical certificate issued. It may take up to 15 years for a company to recover the cost of training a pilot so the long term physical and mental fitness of the applicant must be assured. Thus, what seems to be a small blemish on an otherwise perfect medical record (which still meets the licensing standards of the authority) may result in rejection by the commercial operator: for example, an undescended testicle in childhood may be considered unacceptable, despite successful surgical treatment, because of the slightly increased risk of malignancy.[22] As another example, sick leave

145

TABLE 10.3—Diagnoses incompatible with the issue of a medical certificate by an authorised medical examiner

Cardiovascular disorders	Congenital heart disease Myocardial ischaemia or infarction* Hypertension* Dysrhythmias* Anaemia
Respiratory disorders	Asthma and hay fever (unless mild and controlled)* Pulmonary tuberculosis Spontaneous pneumothorax* Chronic obstructive airways disease Sarcoidosis*
Endocrine disorders	Diabetes mellitus* Other significant endocrine disturbances
Gastrointestinal disorders	Peptic ulcer* Crohn's disease Ulcerative colitis Gallbladder disease
Urogenital disorders	Recurrent calculi Proteinuria
Neurological disorders	Demyelinating disease Epilepsy Migraine (unless infrequent, not incapacitating, and not requiring treatment) Myasthenia gravis Cerebrovascular disease Tertiary syphilis Recent head injury* Unpredictable syncope*
Psychiatric disorders	Neurosis (particularly anxiety, hysteria, phobia, obsession, depression) Personality disorder Dementias Psychoses Alcoholism* and drug abuse
Otolaryngological disorders	Acute or chronic otitis media Hearing loss (beyond Civil Aviation Authority defined limits) Vestibular disease (Menière's, neuronitis, positional vertigo)
Ophthalmic disorders	Visual acuity or colour vision below standards* Uveitis Glaucoma
Other conditions	Most malignancies Hodgkin's disease Gross obesity Orthopaedic problems HIV infection*

*See text.

might have to be taken in the future for a hip replacement because of a traumatic fracture sustained during adolescence.

Although the initial medical examination serves primarily as a selection process, it also has a most important role in providing baseline data against which subsequent information from periodic medical examinations may be compared.

Periodic medical examination

Renewal of a pilot's licence will depend, among other things, on satisfactory medical reassessment at regular statutory intervals which are determined by the class of licence issued and the age of the applicant. Table 10.2 summarises the current intervals between periodic medical examinations and the standards required at each.

By increasing the likelihood of early detection of disease a routine medical examination is regarded as a valuable preventive tool. The yield from periodic medical examinations has, however, been said to be very low, especially in younger age groups: in one report, less than 5% of paired examinations studied showed any positive differences.[23] However, these examinations probably do no harm,[24] and the knowledge that "success" at such reviews is vital to a continued flying career may itself be of value in maintaining health. Furthermore, in the 28 months to December 1976, 58 of the 77 cardiovascular abnormalities that led to loss of licence in the United Kingdom were detected on routine examination.[25] It should also be remembered that pilots are under regular and intense scrutiny—probably more so than any other profession—during, for example, training and regular line flights and simulator checks and as a result some referrals for medical problems in aircrew may come from non-medical sources such as trainers.

Specific medical considerations

No matter how a pilot reaches the doctor's consulting room there are several well recognised areas to which the examining physician must pay particular attention.

Cardiovascular disorders

In civil aviation, cardiovascular disorders are the most common reason for loss or restriction of an aircrew licence. In the United

Kingdom alone, such disorders accounted for about 55% of losses in 1983,[26] and about 41% in the years 1984–1986. Not surprisingly, therefore, an enormous effort is made to establish authoritative guidelines for cardiovascular fitness to fly.

Over the past decade, in a bid to improve the relatively ignorant and largely empirical approach to aviation cardiology previously adopted, a group of British specialists with a professional interest in both cardiovascular and aviation medicine has pioneered new thinking on all aspects of their clinical specialty as it relates to civil aviation and aircrew licensing. The first UK Workshop in Aviation Cardiology was held in July 1982, and the second 5 years later.[27,28] The deliberations of these gatherings produced cardiovascular licensing guidelines which are widely accepted. In October 1991, the first European workshop was convened and took as its agenda items of enduring concern including risk analysis, coronary artery disease, hypertension, and disturbances of conduction and rhythm.[7]

Risk analysis—Air travel is remarkably safe, and it is to the credit of all concerned that of the billions of passengers carried over the past decade, each year an average of just 39 accidents involving scheduled services claimed the lives of 1063 people.[29] These accidents had many causes, including failure of structure, engines or systems, terrorism, aircrew error and aircrew incapacitation, but a reduction in each is being actively pursued. The airworthiness authorities have set a safety target of better than one fatal accident in multicrew aircraft per 10 million flying hours, and it has been suggested that the contribution to this from pilot incapacitation should be better than one fatal accident per 100 million flying hours.[30] This target is considered attainable if the risk to an individual of sudden and complete medical incapacitation in the cockpit is no greater than 1% per year.[31] Acceptance of this approach has led to the adoption of the "1% rule" for cardiovascular risk to pilots in the United Kingdom; a risk equivalent to that of annual cardiovascular mortality in a 65-year-old man. The risk analysis must, however, include all known factors including blood pressure, serum cholesterol, smoking habit, sex, and, importantly, age.[32] No one factor has a fixed and/or sinister significance, and an overall risk must be computed: this aspect has led to much concern over the proposed Joint Aviation Authority regulations in which, for example, a single raised blood cholesterol level could be interpreted and acted upon in isolation.

Coronary artery disease—Coronary artery disease accounts for most of the cardiovascular disorders leading to loss of licence. If the disease is overt there is no dilemma for the licensing authority, but considerable difficulty follows the discovery of asymptomatic electrocardiographic changes on routine examination. Evidence of unequivocal infarction should lead to immediate revocation of the licence but any other changes—for example, ST segment and T wave abnormalities, which are common in normal people—demand referral for further assessment, which will usually require exercise testing perhaps with β blockade. These tests will often correct the ST segment and T wave changes if the myocardium is healthy (although β blockade has also been shown to improve or even return to normal the electrocardiograms of those with ischaemic heart disease[33]). Where doubt remains, exercise ^{201}Tl scintigraphy or echocardiography (or both) may be performed, while coronary angiography may be required in selected cases.[34] The need for such careful assessment, particularly when a professional career is threatened, was amply illustrated in a study in which all but one of 20 asymptomatic subjects with ischaemic changes on electrocardiograms were shown to have unobstructed coronary arteries.[35]

A pilot who presents an only slightly increased overall risk of sudden incapacitation may be allowed to continue flying with or as a copilot because experience has shown the success of mandatory incapacitation training in airline operations. Two pilots with waivers like this must not be rostered to fly together, and so such endorsements do not help flexibility in commercial operations. Follow up exercise electrocardiography or Tl scanning should be undertaken annually.

Advances in the surgical treatment of coronary artery disease have led to the possibility of licence reinstatement following careful postoperative assessment.[36,37] Thus those who have undergone coronary artery bypass grafting or percutaneous transluminal coronary angioplasty may be allowed a restricted (multicrew) licence if, after 9 or 6 months respectively, coronary angiography demonstrates satisfactory circulation. Repeated angiography will be necessary every 2–3 years thereafter. During the years 1984–1991, the United Kingdom Civil Aviation Authority Medical Advisory Panel issued 14 restricted licences (eight class 1 and six class 3) to individuals who had undergone bypass grafting; but four pilots were considered unfit in any licence category.[38]

In military aviation, myocardial infarction results in permanent grounding, whether or not surgery has been undertaken. The rationale for this is that physical and psychological stresses are known to aggravate coronary artery disease, and combat flying is nothing if not stressful. Thus, to the possibly deleterious effects of flight stresses such as hypoxia, acceleration, and thermal strain must be added those of excitement, anxiety, fatigue, and sleep loss during intensive air operations. There is also always a risk that a military aviator will need to cope with ejection and injury, and thereafter with survival in hostile environments (in both the climatic and political sense).

Hypertension—Although the concept of essential hypertension as a quantitative extension of "normotension" is generally appreciated, a precise numerical definition of what is and what is not hypertension is still frequently sought. To this difficulty is added the need to identify those at risk, an identification often based on consulting room measurements of "casual" blood pressure. Because of the serious import for the careers of aviators, the diagnosis of hypertension must be beyond doubt, and Ledingham has suggested that such casual measurements act only as pointers to further assessment. Thus, he recommends that a consulting room blood pressure measurement of $\geqslant 165/90$ mmHg should be followed by ambulatory recordings.[39] Only if average daily ambulatory levels of $\geqslant 150/90$ mmHg are demonstrated should investigation and treatment be triggered. In the presence of endorgan disease, however, even a casual reading of 165/90 mmHg should initiate intervention.

Confirmation of elevated blood pressure requires specialist referral for full investigation, including a thorough clinical search for peripheral vascular disease, electrocardiography, radiography of the renal tract, renal function tests, haematology, and blood biochemistry.

Many non-pharmacological measures have been proposed for the treatment of hypertension, such as weight reduction and exercise, sodium restriction but other elemental supplements (calcium, potassium or magnesium), vegetarian diets, total lipid restriction, reduced alcohol intake, and biofeedback techniques. Long term results of these strategies have been disappointing, however, and their best application is probably as adjuncts to pharmacological therapy, and as the manifestations of a generally healthier lifestyle.[40]

150

Although many antihypertensive drugs are available, the peculiar needs of aircrew mean that not all can be considered for use in this group. Potential side effects such as hypotension, dysrhythmias, depression and drowsiness must all be considered, and the problems of drug interactions may preclude the use of certain combinations. For aircrew, the best policy is to use a single drug if at all possible (monotherapy) even if this means that a trial of several drugs is needed. The chosen drug should then be administered in the lowest effective dose.[41] At present, four classes of antihypertensive drugs can be considered as potentially suitable for aircrew use:

• *β blockers* Cardioselective hydrophilic β-adrenergic blockers such as atenolol, nadolol and sotalol are now the drugs of choice for treatment of aircrew with hypertension, because their side effects, particularly on performance, are minimal. Even so, drowsiness and fatigue, as well as peripheral vascular problems, can and do occur.

• *Diuretics* There remains a place in antihypertensive therapy for the use of diuretics; hydrochlorothiazide (and its derivatives) is the preferred choice because of its smoothness of action and lack of acute side effects. Potassium sparing agents, such as amiloride and triamterene are equally useful alone or in combination with a thiazide, but loop diuretics should be avoided because they may induce hyponatraemic hypotension.

• *Calcium antagonists* The slow channel calcium blocking agents are now regarded as well tolerated and safe, with insignificant central effects, although flushing, headaches and oedema are common especially with the dihydropyridine derivatives such as nifedipine. Combination of this type of drug with a β blocker is therefore recommended. Verapamil and diltiazem are also effective, but should not be used in combination with β blockers.

• *Angiotensin II converting enzyme (ACE) inhibitors* This relatively new group of drugs is also regarded as safe and effective. Longer acting agents such as lisinopril and enalapril are the preferred choice, although captopril may be used. These drugs are especially effective in combination with diuretics (but not with loop agents).

Vasodilator drugs such as hydralazine and dihydralazine should not be used in isolation, but may be very effective when combined with β blockers or ACE inhibitors.[41] Finally, it should be noted that centrally acting antihypertensives (such as reserpine, cloni-dine and methyldopa) and the α-adrenergic blocking agents (such as phentolamine, phenoxybenzamine, and prazosin) are *not* suit-able for aircrew use.

Whatever the chosen therapy, it is essential that an adequate trial of treatment and assessment of side effects is undertaken on the ground before any flying is considered. To that end, a period of compulsory grounding of at least 4 weeks followed by a simulator session or check ride is strongly recommended.[7]

Disturbances of conduction and rhythm—The electrophysiology of cardiac behaviour is extraordinarily complex, and it is not surprising that disturbances of conduction and rhythm require very careful assessment when discovered in an aviator. The success of incapacitation training has, however, meant that conditions previously associated with a bar to future flying are increasingly being considered as compatible with a multicrew restricted licence. During the years 1984–1991, the Civil Aviation Authority's Med-ical Advisory Panel considered a total of 48 cases involving such conditions and granted unrestricted licences to 18 (12 class 1, and six class 3) and restricted licenses to 26 (24 class 1, and two class 3): four cases were found unfit in any category.[38] Table 10.4 summar-ises the advice on disposition offered at the 1991 workshop on aviation cardiology.[7,42-45]

Many drugs are available for the treatment of dysrhythmias but, as with antihypertensives, most are unsuitable for aircrew use because of unacceptable side effects. Thus, only hydrophilic β blocking agents, calcium antagonists such as verapamil, and digi-talis glycosides can be considered for use in this context.[46] This excludes many highly effective agents including all class 1 drugs (for example quinidine, procainamide and disopyramide (1a), mexiletene and diphenylhydantoin (1b), and flecainide (1c)), many class 2 drugs (for example, the lipophilic β blockers), and class 3 drugs (such as amiodarone) except those which also have class 2 actions such as sotalol.

Finally, in the absence of any other disqualifying condition, aircrew deemed to be suitable candidates for cardiac pacing may be given a multicrew restricted licence after a 3 month trial of the pacemaker on the ground. The device should be bipolar, and should be selected from a list of those known to be reliable. Regular (6-monthly) follow up is essential and should include Holter monitoring. Unrestricted licensing is not possible because

TABLE 10.4—Disturbances of conduction and rhythm—general guidelines[42-45]

Abnormality	Licensing	Notes
Sinus node dysfunction	Restricted*	Provided asymptomatic with no organic heart disease, and pauses $\leqslant 2$–2·5 s. Barred if pauses symptomatic
Atrioventricular block		
1st degree (P-R >0·2 s)	Unrestricted†	Provided no bundle branch block present
2nd degree		
Mobitz I	Unrestricted	Provided asymptomatic with no distal block, and intermittent. Barred if bundle branch block present
Mobitz II	Barred	
High grade	Barred	
Congenital complete	Barred	
Intraventricular block		
right bundle branch	Unrestricted	If pre-existing and isolated
	Restricted*	If newly acquired
	Barred	If AV interval prolonged
left bundle branch	Restricted*	Barred if recently acquired
hemiblock	Unrestricted	
Atrial fibrillation		
single isolated (lone)	Restricted*	Following 3–6 months grounding
established	Restricted*	Provided no valve disease or hypertension
paroxysmal	Barred	Unless attacks can be suppressed
chronic	Restricted*	Provided rate is controlled under flight conditions. Barred if on warfarin
Atrial flutter	Barred	
Ventricular ectopics		
unifocal $< 200\,\text{h}^{-1}$	Unrestricted†	Restricted or barred if cardiovascular disease discovered
unifocal $> 200\,\text{h}^{-1}$	Unrestricted†	If invasive assessment normal
Ventricular tachycardia	Restricted*	
($\geqslant 3$ consecutive ectopics at a heart rate $\geqslant 120$)	Barred	If any cardiac abnormality detected
Pre-excitation patterns	Restricted*	

*Restricted refers to multicrew operations only
†Subject to normal exercise electrocardiography and Holter monitoring
  ($\pm$ two-dimensional echocardiography $\pm$ scintigraphy $\pm$ angiography).
  Regular (annual) follow up investigation may be required.

153

of the risks of technical failure and of electromagnetic interference.[47]

Psychiatric disorders

Psychiatric illness is the other major cause of loss of licence: in civil aviation it is second only to cardiovascular disease.[26] Predictably, wastage is highest in the early phases of flying training when the hazards of aviation are new and frightening, but a second peak appears in the fifth and sixth decades. In professional aircrew psychiatric illness is usually related to domestic stress or training problems[48] such as conversion to new types of aircraft. Recognition of the disease state is the most difficult and yet the most important problem facing the authorised medical examiner.

In aircrew, the onset of a neurosis requires immediate grounding, at least for the acute stage and while drugs incompatible with the flying task are being used. A return to flying may be considered if a single episode remits fairly quickly and completely. A protracted illness, or one which relapses, is an indication for permanent loss of licence, as is a neurosis, such as fear of clouds, induced by the stress of flying. The organic components of psychosomatic disorders must be treated appropriately but some—including migraine and asthma for example—may be incompatible with a continued flying career. The development of a functional psychosis requires immediate and permanent withdrawal of a licence as does any episode of drug dependence, but other personality disorders, including alcoholism (see below), may allow continued flying under very close supervision. It is of interest that the Federal Aviation Administration is considering the introduction of a minimental status screening examination as a part of the medical assessment of aircrew, but current techniques are unlikely to be sufficiently sensitive or relevant to achieve the desired aims.[49]

Respiratory disorders

Any respiratory disorder may cause incapacitation in flight and, rarely, death.[50] Thus the risk of stress induced incapacitation as a result of asthma usually means that the onset of this disorder is disqualifying in aircrew. If the sufferer is allowed to continue flying—for example a navigator or engineer with mild illness—limitations are necessary and monitoring must be strict. Treatment with disodium cromoglycate is permissible if it alone is able to suppress symptoms, but this is unusual and the need for antihistamines, steroids, or bronchodilator inhalers leads to grounding.

Recurrence after a first spontaneous pneumothorax is common[51] and because of this increased risk pneumothorax is another condition that leads to immediate suspension of licence. A return to flying may be considered if, 3 months after pleurectomy (preferably bilateral), an attempt to induce an artificial pneumothorax fails. Many thoracic centres and the Royal Air Force have now abandoned the use of chemical pleurodesis because this procedure has been shown to result in a high recurrence rate.[51]

Pulmonary sarcoidosis, a relatively common disorder,[52] is usually discovered on routine chest radiography. When the acute phase has regressed sarcoidosis is compatible with a return to flying duties with adequate supervision. The aeromedical interest shown in this illness in the late 1970s was as a result of its discovery at necropsy in the organs (and particularly the myocardium) of several aircrew who were in aircraft accidents. The finding was considered to be incidental, but concern remains with regard to the rare possibility of sudden incapacitation due to cardiac involvement: full cardiovascular assessment has been recommended in all patients with sarcoidosis before returning to flying duties. In those with isolated hilar but no systemic involvement, a restricted licence may be granted provided that the resting, exercise, and ambulatory electrocardiograms are normal and a ^{201}Tl scan is also satisfactory. Those with systemic sarcoidosis but with normal lung function, no requirement for steroid therapy, and with no demonstrable cardiac involvement are also eligible for a restricted licence, but will require 6-monthly review. Should cardiac involvement be demonstrated, however, immediate loss of licence is mandatory.[53]

Endocrine disorders

International Civil Aviation Organization guidelines allow professional aircrew who develop diabetes mellitus to continue flying provided that good control can be achieved by diet alone. Private pilots and air traffic control officers may also be relicensed if they are sufficiently well controlled on a biguanide oral hypoglycaemic agent. All diabetic aviators, however, must achieve satisfactory medical results at frequent intervals if they are to retain their licences. Thus body weight must be shown to be constant, the 2-hour postprandial blood sugar concentration must be less than $8.25 \, \mathrm{mmol} \, l^{-1}$ ($150 \, \mathrm{mg} \, 100 \, \mathrm{ml}^{-1}$) and the urine must be free of protein and ketones with only a trace of sugar allowed. Furthermore, electrocardiographic, blood pressure, visual function, and central and peripheral neurological examinations must be normal. Such rigorous requirements are difficult to maintain.

Other conditions

Obesity—Acquired major obesity is uncommon in aircrew, who have a high motivation to remain flying: any increase in weight is usually recognised early and dealt with appropriately.

Peptic ulceration—The development of peptic ulcer in experienced aircrew leads to grounding for the initial treatment phase and the presence or absence of complications will determine any resumption of flying. Surgery should be considered early in cases which bleed, or following two relapses after medical treatment.

Neurological disorders—Neurological disorders such as degenerative or neurovascular diseases, neuralgias, tumours, dementias, and multiple sclerosis are all permanent bars, but inflammations and head injuries may allow a return to flying. On-the-job performance testing may be required.

In the case of a closed head injury further guidelines are laid down because the degree of post-traumatic amnesia is a reasonable indication of the extent of brain damage, and hence of the subsequent development of post-traumatic epilepsy.[54] Thus, a permanent bar is imposed if the duration of amnesia is longer than 4 weeks, or if there is permanent loss of cerebral function. Amnesia of 3, 2, or 1 week's duration is followed by grounding for 12, 9, or 6 months respectively, while a transient amnesia requires grounding for at least 6 weeks.

Other causes of disturbance of consciousness—such as hyperglycaemia or hypoglycaemia, fugues, cerebrovascular accidents, vertigo, and simple faints—require full investigation, and only a confirmed, simple, predictable, explicable, and therefore preventable vasovagal syncope would be compatible with a return to a full flying category.

Finally, for the reasons discussed above, a diagnosis of HIV positivity should lead to an immediate and irrevocable bar to further licensing.

The female pilot

Female aircrew have been a part of the civilian aviation environment for many years and, while various studies have been conducted on the possible effects of flight upon female physiology, it is generally held that under normal circumstances there are no significant differences between the sexes with regard to the skills and attributes needed to operate a commercial aircraft. (It is interesting to note that it has taken 30 years for a woman to be appointed a pilot of concorde: the reasons for this may be many and varied, but they will not include any aeromedical considerations.) Pregnancy is not, however, a normal circumstance in this context, and menstruation may not be.

Pregnancy brings with it a host of physiological changes, many of which (including haemodynamic changes, hyperventilation, and vasomotor rhinitis) could affect tolerance to the flight environment.[55] If a pregnant woman applies for a pilot's licence, current International Civil Aviation Organization guidelines are that the application should be temporarily refused, while pregnant women already holding a licence should not be permitted to fly until the second trimester, and only then as part of a multicrew. Commercial interests dictate that flying as a pilot at any stage of a declared pregnancy is unlikely to be allowed.

The possible association of menstruation with decrements in performance has been the subject of many studies of the perimenstrual phase compared with the rest of the cycle. The majority, however, have concluded that neither cognitive nor motor performance is adversely affected by the cyclical hormonal fluctuations or mood swings of a normal oestrous cycle. Accordingly, "... it seems unlikely that fluctuations in performance due to premenstrual tension would have a detectable general effect on flight safety."[56]

Although women have also been employed in military aviation for many decades, it is only within the last few years that all flying roles, including combat, have been open to them. In a recent wide ranging review of women in the military fast jet role, Lyons[57] has determined that in this environment too there are only minor differences between the sexes. Lyons examined ergonomic and related issues such as anatomy and physiology, anthropometry, aerobic fitness and strength; aeromedical issues such as the response to acceleration, altitude and pressure changes, and temperature extremes; and clinical issues such as illness and injury, and pregnancy. He concluded that anatomy and physiology "present no insurmountable problems to women participating in military aviation". Those difficulties which exist in the areas of anthropometry, fitness and strength are such that engineering solutions are possible if there is political will and economic wherewithal. And, while women may be more susceptible than men to motion sickness, radiation induced cancers, and decompression illness, they may be more resistant to cold water immersion and chronic hypoxia (altitude sickness). Tolerance to acute hypoxia is the same for men and women. Furthermore, differences between the sexes in work performance, acceleration tolerance, heat stress, and injury rate are insignificant when size, strength and fitness are balanced.

Only the potential dangers to the fetus in the early stages of an undiagnosed pregnancy give rise to anxiety, and even here the only strong evidence is that suggesting radiation damage because of exposure to high altitude. Other unproven hazards to the embryo include heat stress, acceleration, decompression, noise, and vibration. Concern over these risks during high altitude flying led the United States Air Force Strategic Air Command Scientific Advisory Board to recommend contraception, with pregnancy testing every 14 days.[58]

The ageing pilot

The problems associated with ageing must be recognised when aircrew are in their fifth decade and beyond. Such problems include not only the well known increases in the risk of hypertension and ischaemic heart disease but also the increasing difficulty in coping with irregular work and sleep, the increasing likelihood of functional psychoses, and the degradation of auditory and visual functions. The increased frequency of periodic medical examinations with age is the means by which most of these problems are monitored, but the way in which various functions are assessed could probably be improved. For example, one review has suggested that current tests of visual ability should be supplemented with tests more relevant to pilot performance such as contrast sensitivity, function in low light levels, and dynamic visual acuity.[59]

Medication

Because of the problems that may result from loss of licence, aircrew may not declare a history of illness at medical examinations, even though this information is actively sought by a written questionnaire at each medical. Because the medical examiner is often not the pilot's usual doctor, great reliance is placed on the integrity of the examinee. Under certain circumstances aircrew may also be tempted to seek treatment from a private practitioner in the belief that medical information will not be passed back to medical examiners or the licensing authority.

The question of whether a doctor should automatically inform the authority of illnesses that are potentially lethal (to others) is a vexed one that is inevitably complicated by the ethical position of the doctor in relation to a patient. In this context, the advice long offered to doctors when dealing with similar dilemmas on the ground is most apposite: "... rarely, the public interest may persuade the doctor that his duty to the community may override his duty to maintain his patient's confidence ..."[60] Failure to report such cases may have disastrous consequences, as illustrated by the notorious 1966 Lockheed Electra accident in the United States which resulted in the loss of 83 lives. The probable cause of this accident was pilot incapacitation caused by coronary insufficiency at a critical phase of landing. Subsequent investigation showed that for some years the pilot had been receiving treatment for angina pectoris and diabetes mellitus, but had not declared this history to his aviation medical examiner.[61]

Before any medication is prescribed for aircrew the doctor must be satisfied that both the condition and the proposed treatment are not contraindications to flight. For example, blurring of vision caused by anticholinergic drugs is an unacceptable side effect, as would be any adverse effect on mental performance. In addition, the possibility of hypersensitivity or idiosyncratic reactions must be assessed by a trial of the drug on the ground for at least 24 hours before flight.

Hypnotics—Irregularities in work and rest created by airline operations are such that aircrew may seek medical advice and a prescription for hypnotics. In general practice the benzodiazepines have been established as "first line" treatment because of their efficacy and relative safety, but they have also been shown to have deleterious effects on mental performance.[62,63] Some benzodiazepines have long elimination half lives—for example, 14–90 hours for diazepam—which can produce accumulation and so prolong adverse effects on performance,[64] so that daily use in aircrew should be avoided. Furthermore, because prolonged use of benzodiazepines may also result in dependence[65] the choice of such drugs for use by aircrew must be made with care. They should certainly

159

be prescribed at the lowest dose possible and should have been tried on the ground before operational use. An interval of 24 hours between ingestion and duty should be set, and the pilot should abstain from alcohol because it may have a synergistic rather than a simple additive effect on performance when combined with a benzodiazepine.[66] Temazepam is probably the hypnotic of choice and was used extensively with success by British military aircrew during the Falklands conflict.[67] Other psychotropic drugs should be given only to grounded aircrew, not only because they are likely to compromise performance[68] but also because the conditions for which they are prescribed are usually incompatible with flying duties.

Antihistamines—Antihistamines (H$_1$ receptor antagonists) should not be prescribed, except in topical preparations, because they may produce sedation and impairment of performance at therapeutic dosage.[69] Self medication may, however, occur because they are often incorporated into products that are bought "over the counter". In a 1982 United States Navy accident, which resulted in 14 deaths, the pilot's use of a proprietory cold cure was listed as a contributory factor to the cause of the accident.[70] At necropsy, his blood contained brompheniramine (an antihistamine known to impair performance[71]) at 6–11 times the normal therapeutic range. The development of two antihistamines, astemizole and terfenadine, which are apparently free of sedative side effects at therapeutic concentrations,[69,72] is only a partial solution, because the conditions for which antihistamines are commonly prescribed may not be compatible with flight. This is also true of H$_2$ receptor antagonists prescribed for the treatment of peptic ulcer.

Steroids and antibiotics—The possibility that flying will be contraindicated by the diagnosed condition usually excludes the use of steroids and antibiotics in operational aircrew. Long term antibiotic treatment may occasionally be required in conditions compatible with flying—for example in acne or prolonged episodes of nonspecific urethritis. Most antibiotics are intrinsically safe when used in otherwise healthy people, but possible hypersensitivity must always be excluded by a trial on the ground. The aminoglycosides should, however, be avoided because of the risk of damage to the vestibular nerve which, although rare, would have serious consequences for a pilot's career. On the whole, the decision to prescribe medication to aircrew must be based on sound clinical pharmacology applied with medical common sense and helped by a basic understanding of the aviation environment. The only occasion when medication *must* be given to all aircrew is when they are likely to enter a malarial area. All antimalarials at present used for prophylaxis are safe for use in aircrew, and the choice of agent will be determined by the current pattern of drug resistance. Information on this is available from the Public Health Laboratory Service.[73] Finally, concerned by the apparent failure of its aircrew to comply with antimalaria regimes, British Airways now issues its long haul crews with treatment packs containing diagnostic equipment and halofantrine which, it is hoped, will raise the index of suspicion both among staff and the doctors they consult, and thereby encourage timely diagnosis.

Self medication and alcohol

In some parts of the world it is legal to purchase medicines which in the United Kingdom would be available only on prescription. As a result, aircrew are constantly warned to avoid self medication, and that availability does not necessarily equate with safety. Especial care must be exercised with cold cures (see above) and antidiarrhoea agents which may contain opiates or anticholinergics. Nevertheless, the relevance of drugs to aviation accidents has necessitated the development of comprehensive toxicological screening procedures which use extraction techniques of sufficient efficiency to allow the sensitive detection of even subtherapeutic concentrations of drugs at necropsy.[74] In a survey of toxicological examinations made on 1345 pilots killed in American general aviation during a 7 year period (1968–74) drugs were identified in 16 (1–2%) cases, but this percentage was small compared with the presence of alcohol in 262 (19·5%) pilots. Of these cases, the blood alcohol concentration in 117 (8·7% of the total) was in excess of 0·05%, a concentration high enough to be a possible contributing factor to an accident.[75] More recently, in a similar study of 294 cases from the United States Air Force, of the 196 fatalities 43 (22%) were positive for toxicology, 14 (7%) had positive drug analyses (cold cures and antimalarial drugs), and alcohol (probably post mortem) was identified in 9 (4·6%). Corresponding figures for the 98 nonfatal cases were 14, six and nil respectively.[76] In general aviation, it is estimated that alcohol is present in the blood and tissues of 10–30% of those involved in fatal accidents due to pilot error, although in military and commercial aviation alcohol is implicated in very few fatal accidents.[77]

161

The adverse effects of alcohol on judgement and the performance of skilled tasks have long been recognised by the airlines, who frequently recommend a minimum period of 8–12 hours "from bottle-to-throttle" for their aircrew. In the mid 1980s, the Federal Aviation Administration implemented regulations which forbad operation, or attempted operation, of a civil aircraft by anyone within 8 hours of consuming any alcoholic beverage. It was also ruled that to operate an aircraft with a blood alcohol level in excess of 8.7 mmol l^{-1} (0.04% by weight) was an offence. In practice, the 8-hour interval may be too short because the rate of removal of alcohol from blood is relatively slow—about 3.26 mmol l^{-1} h^{-1} or 8 g h^{-1}.[78] A rule based on time alone may therefore be ineffective unless defined limits are also applied to the quantity of alcohol consumed. So, for example, if a "standard" drink is taken to be 44 ml of spirits, 360 ml of beer, or 150 ml of wine, each of which contains about 15 g of alcohol,[77] detectable blood concentrations may still be present over 8 hours after the ingestion of just 4 pints of beer.

Alcohol abuse is increasing in the United Kingdom and there is no reason to suppose that aircrew are any less susceptible to this problem than their non-flying peers. A retrospective analysis of liver histology from 423 United Kingdom aircrew (of all types) killed in aviation accidents between 1955 and 1979 suggested that 19 (4.5%) had histopathological evidence of alcohol abuse.[79] In the United States, a survey of 1169 private and professional pilots revealed that 16% could be regarded as heavy drinkers (that is, more than five "standard" drinks per occasion twice monthly, or an average of more than two drinks per day).[80] Although these figures are unlikely to represent a higher incidence than that of any similar socioeconomic group, the nature of a pilot's occupation must make detection of this problem a priority, especially as self-confession is rare. Blood sampling for γ-glutamyltransferase activity at routine medical examination has often been advocated, but licensing authorities worldwide have concluded that this would not be cost effective, primarily because commercial aircraft accidents rarely have alcohol abuse cited as even a contributory cause. Although alcohol related accidents are more common in private aviation, they are still only a very small proportion—most accidents to private aviators are the result of poor flying technique—and it is not thought that occasional blood tests at routine examination would be an effective deterrent. Testing for alcohol is limited to investigations following accidents, or if there is a reasonable suspicion of alcohol use.

In 1990, in a somewhat bizarre although possibly portentous move, the Federal Aviation Administration implemented mandatory testing for illicit drugs in all flight crew, flight attendants, air and ground dispatchers, aircraft maintenance workers, and air traffic controllers involved in air transportation within the United States.[77] Pilots in general aviation will also be included in this scheme in due course, but private pilots will not. Tests for amphetamines, cocaine, phencyclidine, and tetrahydrocannabinol (a marijuana metabolite) are to be carried out before employment, after an accident, whenever there is reasonable cause, and at random. Tests for alcohol and benzodiazepines, however, are not included; although the former is now the subject of a proposed Federal Aviation Administration rule. The appropriateness of this new scheme has, therefore, been widely challenged, especially because the use of illicit drugs has never been cited as a contributory cause of any major airline accident in the United States, and even in fatal general aviation accidents it is implicated in just 1–2% (cf. alcohol). As an alternative strategy, it has been recommended that the more important problems of alcohol use by aircrew be addressed by an immediate reduction in the allowable blood alcohol to zero, by increasing "bottle-to-throttle" time to 12 hours (and to 24 hours if more than five "standard" drinks have been consumed), and by increasing pilot awareness of the subject by education.[77]

In the meantime, some authorities have instituted biochemical screening for aircrew as a means of both detecting subclinical illness and increasing safety in the air. In 1983, the Icelandic Civil Aviation Administration began extensive testing (at least biennially) of all its flight deck crew and air traffic controllers: an all male, largely middle aged, population of about 352.[81] Full haematological and biochemical analysis is undertaken, including haemoglobin, haematocrit, mean corpuscular volume, white cell count, erythrocyte sedimentation rate, etc, and serum creatinine, cholesterol, triglycerides, and liver enzymes (aspartate aminotransferase (serum glutamic-oxaloacetic transaminase), alanine aminotransferase (serum glutamic-pyruvic transaminase), *and* γ-glutamyl transferase). In the first few years of this scheme, haematological indices were unremarkable but the biochemical results revealed subclinical diabetes in 15 patients and hyperlipidaemia in 48. In 50 cases, the initial γ-glutamyl transferase was $> 50 \text{ IU l}^{-1}$, a level used to trigger intervention by means of counselling, and in three cases referral to an alcohol treatment unit. In all 50, there was an abrupt fall in the level of this enzyme when next measured.

Once a diagnosis of alcoholism has been made, loss of licence is automatic but the alcoholic pilot may be reinstated if clinical evidence of recovery, including a 2 year period of abstinence, is established.

Conclusion

Determination of crew fitness to fly is an important and sometimes difficult task which embraces all aspects of clinical and preventive medicine. Examining doctors must be aware of the many nuances surrounding the unique environment (the cockpit) in which their patients work, and of the responsibilities they hold not only for the wellbeing of those patients, but also for that of passengers and the public at large.

1 Harper CR, Kidera GJ, Cullen JF. Study of simulated airline pilot incapacitation: phase II subtle or partial loss of function. *Aerospace Med* 1971; **42**: 946–8.
2 Buley LE. Incidence, causes and results of airline pilot incapacitation while on duty. *Aerospace Med* 1969; **40**: 64–70.
3 James M, Green R. Airline pilot incapacitation survey. *Aviat Space Environ Med* 1991; **62**: 1068–72.
4 Martin-Saint-Laurent A, Lavernhe MD, Casano G, Simkoff A. Clinical aspects of inflight incapacitations in commercial aviation. *Aviat Space Environ Med* 1990; **61**: 256–60.
5 Bennett G. Pilot incapacitation and aircraft accidents. *Eur Heart J* 1988; **9** (suppl. G): 21–4.
6 Booze CF. Sudden inflight incapacitation in general aviation. *Aviat Space Environ Med* 1989; **60**: 332–5.
7 Joy M. Introduction and summary of principal conclusions to the first european workshop in aviation cardiology. *Eur Heart J* 1992; **13** (suppl. H): 1–9.
8 International Civil Aviation Organization. *Manual of civil aviation medicine*, 2nd edn. Montreal: ICAO, 1985.
9 Anonymous. New flightcrew licensing rules delayed. *Flight International* 1993; **143** (Number 4361): 6.
10 Beers KN, Mohler SR. The new FAA national automated ECG network: some aviation medical examiner experiences. *Aviat Space Environ Med* 1991; **62**: 62–6.
11 Piepgrass SR, Uhl GS, Hickman JR, Hopkirk JAC, Plowman K. Limitations of the exercise stress test in the detection of coronary artery disease in apparently healthy men. *Aviat Space Environ Med* 1982; **53**: 379–82.
12 Bruce RA. Values and limitations of exercise electrocardiography (editorial). *Circulation* 1974; **50**: 1–3.
13 Broustet JP, Douard H, Oysel N, Rougier P, Koch M. What is the predictive value of exercise electrocardiography in the investigation of male aircrew aged 40–60 years old? *Eur Heart J* 1992; **13** (suppl. H): 59–69.
14 Fuchs HS. Hypertension and orthostatic hypotension in applicants for flying training and aircrew. *Aviat Space Environ Med* 1983; **54**: 65–8.
15 Aerospace Medical Association Special Committee Report. HIV positivity and aviation safety. *Aviat Space Environ Med* 1992; **63**: 375–7.
16 AsMA policy statement on HIV-infected pilots. *Aviat Space Environ Med* 1991; **62**: 1012.

17 Clark JB. Policy considerations of human immunodeficiency virus (HIV) infection in US naval aviation personnel. *Aviat Space Environ Med* 1990; **61:** 165–8.

18 Selnes OA, Miller EN. Asymptomatic HIV-1 infection and aviation safety (letters to the Editor). *Aviat Space Environ Med* 1993; **64:** 172–5.

19 World Health Organization. *Report of the consultation on the neuropsychiatric aspects of HIV infection.* Geneva: World Health Organization, 1988.

20 World Health Organization. *Report of the second consultation on the neuropsychiatric aspects of HIV-1 infection.* Geneva: World Health Organization, 1990.

21 Department of Health. *Immunization against infectious disease.* London: HMSO, 1992: 9.

22 Rains AJH, Capper WM. *Bailey and Love's short practice of surgery*, 15th edn. London: Lewis, 1971: 1242.

23 Rossing RG, Allen MF. Information yield of the annual medical examination for flying. *Aerospace Med* 1973; **44:** 936–43.

24 Anonymous. Routine medical examinations (editorial). *Lancet* 1969; **ii:** 833.

25 Joy MD. The impact of coronary vascular risk factors on professional aircrew licence loss in the UK. Specific findings in cardiac and pulmonary function with special emphasis on assessment criteria for flying. *AGARD conference proceedings 232.* Neuilly-sur-Seine, France: NATO Advisory Group for Research and Development, 1977: B19.1–B19.6.

26 Bennett G. Psychiatric disorders in civilian pilots. *Aviat Space Environ Med* 1983; **54:** 588–9.

27 The First United Kingdom Workshop in Aviation Cardiology. *Eur Heart J* 1984; 5 (suppl. A): 1–164.

28 The Second United Kingdom Workshop in Aviation Cardiology. *Eur Heart J* 1988; 9 (suppl. G): 1–179.

29 Learmount D. Not under control. *Flight International* 1993; **143** (Number 4354): 27–34.

30 Bennett G. Medical cause accidents in commercial aviation. *Eur Heart J* 1992; 13 (suppl. H): 13–15.

31 Tunstall-Pedoe H. The concept of risk. *Eur Heart J* 1988; 9 (suppl. G): 13–15.

32 Tunstall-Pedoe H. Cardiovascular risk and risk factors in the context of aircrew certification. *Eur Heart J* 1992; 13 (suppl. H): 16–20.

33 Prichard BNC. Beta blockade and the effects of stress on the normal and ischaemic heart. *Aviat Space Environ Med* 1981; **52:** S9–S18.

34 Royal College of Physicians of London. The cardiovascular fitness of airline pilots. Report of a working party of the cardiology committee of the Royal College of Physicians of London. *Br Heart J* 1978; **40:** 335–50.

35 Taggart P, Carruthers M, Joseph S *et al.* Electrocardiographic changes resembling myocardial ischaemia in asymptomatic men with normal coronary arteriograms. *Br Heart J* 1979; **41:** 214–25.

36 Dargie HJ. Late results following coronary artery bypass grafting. *Eur Heart J* 1992; 13 (suppl. H): 89–95.

37 Serruys PW, Breeman A. Coronary angioplasty—long-term follow-up results and detection of restenosis: guidelines for aviation cardiology. *Eur Heart J* 1992; 13 (suppl. H): 76–88.

38 Joy M. Cardiological aspects of aviation safety—the new european perspective. *Eur Heart J* 1992; 13 (suppl. H): 21–6.

39 Ledingham JGG. Definitions of hypertension in relation to risk: the role of ambulatory monitoring. *Eur Heart J* 1992; 13 (suppl. H): 35–8.

40 Swales JD. Non-pharmacological antihypertensive therapy. *Eur Heart J* 1988; 9 (suppl. G): 45–52.

41 Brunner HR, Waeber B, Nussberger J. Strategies for the management of hypertension in aircrew. *Eur Heart J* 1992; 13 (suppl. H): 45–9.

42 Rowland E, Morgado F. Sino-atrial node dysfunction, atrioventricular block and intraventricular conduction disturbances. *Eur Heart J* 1992; 13 (suppl. H): 130–5.

43 Kulbertus HE. Implications of lone atrial fibrillation/flutter in the context of cardiovascular fitness to fly. *Eur Heart J* 1992; 13 (suppl. H): 136–8.

44 Campbell RWF. Ventricular rhythm disturbances in the normal heart. *Eur Heart J* 1992; 13 (suppl. H): 139–43.

45 Toff WD, Camm AJ. Ventricular pre-excitation and professional aircrew licensing. *Eur Heart J* 1992; 13 (suppl. H): 149–61.

46 Gorgels APM, Wellens HJJ, Vos MA. Aviation and antiarrhythmic medication. *Eur Heart J* 1992; 13 (suppl. H): 144–8.

165

47 Toff WD, Edhag OK, Camm AJ. Cardiac pacing and aviation. *Eur Heart J* 1992; **13** (suppl. H): 162–75.
48 Bennett G, O'Connor PJ. Medical wastage of military and civil aircrew in Great Britain 1963–1968. *Aerospace Med* 1970; **41:** 550–2.
49 Banich MT, Stokes A, Elledge VC. Neuropsychological screening of aviators: a review. *Aviat Space Environ Med* 1989; **60:** 361–6.
50 Hill IR. Sarcoidosis: a review of some features of importance in aviation medicine. *Aviat Space Environ Med* 1977; **48:** 953–4.
51 Hopkirk JAC, Pullen MJ, Fraser JR. Pleurodesis: the results of treatment for spontaneous pneumothorax in the Royal Air Force. *Aviat Space Environ Med* 1983; **54:** 158–60.
52 Pettyjohn FS, Spoor DH, Buckendorf WA. Sarcoid and the heart—an aeromedical risk. *Aviat Space Environ Med* 1977; **48:** 95–8.
53 Swanton RH. Sarcoidosis of the heart. *Eur Heart J* 1988; **9** (suppl. G): 169–74.
54 Merry RTG. Neurology. In: Ernsting J, King PF, eds. *Aviation medicine*, 2nd edn. London: Butterworths, 1988: 646.
55 Nicholson PJ. Pregnancy and vocational flying. *Travel Med Int* 1992; **10:** 105–8.
56 Smith PR, Chappelow JW. The menstrual cycle and performance. *RAF IAM Report* No 743, March 1993.
57 Lyons TJ. Women in the fast jet cockpit—aeromedical considerations. *Aviat Space Environ Med* 1992; **63:** 809–18.
58 Strategic Air Command Scientific Advisory Board. Medical aspects of the integration of female pilots into U-2/TR-1 aircraft. Headquarters Strategic Air Command, Offutt AFB, Nebraska, 1989.
59 Sekuler R, Kline D, Dismukes K. Aging and visual function of military pilots: a review. *Aviat Space Environ Med* 1982; **53:** 747–58.
60 Raffle A, ed. *Medical aspects of fitness to drive—a guide for medical practitioners*, 3rd edn. London: Medical Commission on Accident Prevention, 1976: 70.
61 Reighard HL, Mohler SR. Some aspects of sudden incapacitation due to cardiovascular disease. *Aerospace Med* 1967; **38:** 1273–5.
62 McNair DM. Anti-anxiety drugs and human performance. *Arch Gen Psychiatry* 1973; **29:** 609–17.
63 Borland RG, Nicholson AN. Comparison of the residual effects of two benzodiazepines (nitrazepam and flurazepam hydrochloride) and pentobarbitone sodium on human performance. *Br J Clin Pharmacol* 1975; **2:** 9–17.
64 Nicholson AN, Stone BM. *Handbook for flight medical officers.* AGARDograph No 270(E). 2nd ed. Neuilly-sur-Seine, France: NATO Advisory Group for Aerospace Research and Development, 1987.
65 Petursson H, Lader MH. Withdrawal from long-term benzodiazepine treatment. *BMJ* 1981; **283:** 643–5.
66 Subhan Z, Hindmarch I. The effects of midazolam in conjunction with alcohol on iconic memory and recall. *Neuropsychobiology* 1983; **9:** 230–4.
67 Baird JA, Coles PK, Nicholson AN. Human factors and air operations in the south Atlantic campaign: discussion paper. *J R Soc Med* 1983; **76:** 933–7.
68 Snaith RP, Hindmarch I, Standing VF. Psychotropic drugs and road accidents. *BMJ* 1977; **2:** 263.
69 Clarke CH, Nicholson AN. Performance studies with antihistamines. *Br J Clin Pharmacol* 1978; **6:** 31–5.
70 Clausen P. EA-6B Crash on Nimitz attributed to pilot error. *Aviation Weekly and Space Technology* 1982; **117:** 22–3.
71 Nicholson AN. Effect of the antihistamines, brompheniramine maleate and triprolidine hydrochloride, on performance in man. *Br J Clin Pharmacol* 1979; **8:** 321–4.
72 Nicholson AN, Stone BM. Performance studies in man with H_1-histamine receptor antagonists, astemizole and terfenadine. *Br J Clin Pharmacol* 1982; **13:** 199–202.
73 Public Health Laboratory Service Malaria Reference Laboratory. Malaria prophylaxis. *BMJ* 1983; **286:** 787–9.
74 Mayes RW. The extraction and identification of drugs in aviation toxicology. *Aviat Space Environ Med* 1982; **53:** 332–5.
75 Lacefield DJ, Roberts PA, Blossom CW. Toxicological findings in fatal civil aviation accidents, fiscal years 1968–1974. *Aviat Space Environ Med* 1975; **46:** 1030–2.
76 Ruehle CJ. Toxicologic studies on USAF aircraft accident casualties, 1973–1984. *Aviat Space Environ Med* 1989; **60** (suppl. 10): B86–8.

77 Modell JG, Mountz JM. Drinking and flying—the problem of alcohol use by pilots. *New Engl J Med* 1990; **323:** 455–61.
78 Saunders JB, Paton A. ABC of alcohol: alcohol in the body. *BMJ* 1981; **283:** 1380–1.
79 Underwood-Ground KE. Liver pathology in aircrew. *Aviat Space Environ Med* 1982; **53:** 14–18.
80 Ross LE, Ross SM. Pilots' attitudes toward alcohol use and flying. *Aviat Space Environ Med* 1988; **59:** 913–19.
81 Hardarson T, Thordarson U, Arnarson EÖ, Franzon L. Biochemical screening of airmen. *Aviat Space Environ Med* 1988; **59:** 965–7.

11
Special forms of flight

Engines for flying, a man sitting in the midst thereof, by turning onely about an Instrument, which moves artificiall Wings made to beat the Aire, much after the fashion of a Bird's flight.

Roger Bacon (*c.* 1214–1294)

Humans have always sought to emulate the flight of birds, and the ubiquity of modern aviation is evidence of their success. This chapter and the next deal with the aviation medicine aspects of some of the more esoteric forms of human flight.

Balloons

The Montgolfier brothers first demonstrated to the world that human-carrying "engines for flying" were possible 210 years ago. Their vehicle, however, did not have "artificiall Wings" but was a balloon filled with hot air. (A Brazilian, Bartolomeu de Gusmao, had flown a small unmanned hot air balloon in 1709.[1]) After successful unmanned demonstrations, the first recorded human free flight took place on 21 November 1783, when Jean-Francois Pilatre de Rozier, a doctor, and François Laurent, Marquis d'Arlandes, undertook a 25-min flight over Paris in a Montgolfier balloon (in contrast to a Charlier balloon, which is one filled with a gas that is lighter than air and also flew, manned, in the same year).[2] Since that auspicious beginning humans have landed on the moon and sent machines to other planets. Non-powered balloon flight has played a vital part in this amazing advance and still retains a place of its own in modern aviation.

Notwithstanding Pilatre de Rozier's contribution, the history of aviation medicine can truly be said to have begun in 1875. In that year—again in France—a balloon flight to 8784 m (28 820 ft) by three young scientists, Croce-Spenelli, Sivel, and Tissandier, ended in tragedy when they failed to use their oxygen equipment properly.[3] Only Tissandier survived, the others becoming the first victims of aviation hypoxia. Subsequent ascents over the next 60 years showed conclusively—and again sometimes tragically—that flights above about 12 802 m (42 000 ft) were not possible, even when breathing 100% oxygen: the risks and limitations imposed by lack of oxygen, and also by the extreme cold of altitude, were overwhelming.[2] The solution to these two problems, and thus the possibility of higher flights, was pioneered by Auguste Piccard, who in 1931 designed, built, and flew the first ever pressurised cabin—suspended beneath a gas filled balloon—to an altitude of 15 781 m (51 762 ft).[2] The gondola was pressurised to one atmosphere and had its own oxygen supply and a means of eliminating carbon dioxide. Temperature was controlled in later flights by painting the top of the gondola white and the underneath black. This created an acceptable internal temperature of 19·4 °C when the outside temperature was − 55 °C. A similar colour scheme was adopted in the extant high altitude record ascent to 34 656 m (113 700 ft) by Ross and Prather in 1961. On this occasion thermal control was achieved by alternating the exposure of black and silver (aluminium) venetian blinds.[4] The problem of direct and excessive solar heating of objects within enclosed capsules was overcome in the Apollo space programme by slowly rotating the space craft about its longitudinal axis—so-called passive thermal control.[2]

After Piccard's breakthrough, larger gas filled balloons capable of flying to altitudes beyond 30 480 m (100 000 ft) were developed—mainly by American and Soviet military organisations—to test and prove a variety of equipment for future human space programmes. Researching ballooning of this type is now limited, although high altitude unmanned balloons continue to provide vital physical and meteorological information.

Nearer to earth, hot air sport ballooning in open gondolas is a popular and growing activity stemming from the development in the 1950s of new lightweight materials and of balloons equipped with propane gas burners (lighter than air gas balloons are seldom used for sport). Although this sport usually takes place at relatively low altitudes, and everyday minor injuries such as bumped heads and burns from the propane gas systems are fairly common, the major medical problems facing today's balloonists are the same as those encountered by the pioneers of the past: cold and lack of oxygen. Thus any flights above 3048 m (10 000 ft)—such as

169

altitude record attempts or during mountain balloon meets—are clearly those for which expert advice on oxygen equipment and thermal comfort should be obtained. Simple oxygen systems are available which will provide adequate protection up to an altitude of 7620 m (25 000 ft), and protective clothing such as that worn for skiing is recommended. Those who wish to go higher than this run the additional major risk of decompression sickness and again should seek expert advice before flight.

Hot air ballooning has proved to be exceptionally safe; in recent years there have been no fatal accidents in Britain. This probably reflects the high professional and medical standards required of balloon pilots, who are expected by the Civil Aviation Authority to hold a pilot's licence and a medical certificate.

Gliders

Gliders are non-powered craft which are heavier than air and capable of sustained flight. Since their first use in the 1890s their design and performance have been progressively improved, and they have been used extensively—particularly in the past 50 years—for aeronautical and meteorological research, and during the second world war as troop transports. Today they are most often flown for sport, and there are well over 123 000 devotees worldwide.[5]

The Civil Aviation Authority does not require glider pilots to have either a pilot's licence or a medical certificate (although flying instructors and the pilots of motor gliders must have a licence), despite their susceptibility to many of the medical and safety problems that beset their powered colleagues (such as problems of altitude, cockpit workload, and in particular altered perception). For example, difficulties of lookout are exacerbated in the often very crowded thermals over popular gliding sites. This, combined with the problem of internal reflections from the highly curved cockpit transparency, adds to the pilot's visual workload. At sites where high altitude gliding can be achieved, freezing expirate on the canopy may further impair vision. In addition, the constant turning in often turbulent thermals is a strong stimulus for motion sickness, particularly in students and casual passengers. The natural tendency to dehydrate during long flights (compounded by the lack of storage space for food and liquid) can lead to problems at the most critical stage of a flight: the landing. Most of these aspects are given scant attention by many instructors, and only relatively recently has any advice been available in gliding magazines.[6-8] In a relatively recent change for the better the sport's governing body, the British Gliding Association, now lists the use of oxygen as a "recommended practice", and states that oxygen should be carried during flights above 3656 m (12 000 ft). Carrying parachutes is also a "recommended practice".[9] The sport continues to attract criticism from knowledgeable experts over its lack of attention to such matters, and even in the 1990s one reputable gliding journal was promoting the use of archaic oxygen equipment as "the most efficient way known by respiratory physiologist (*sic*) for saturating the blood to over 90%".[10]

The problems of restraint and protection from impact, however, are those most obviously connected with gliding safety. The Civil Aviation Authority no longer provides statistical information on gliding accidents in its annual returns, relying instead on the extensive annual register of accidents and incidents compiled by the British Gliding Association itself.[11] In 1992, for example, the Association reported 145 "assessable" (for cause) accidents involving gliders on the British register, resulting in three fatalities (in 1991 there were seven fatalities).[11,12] The Association has identified an increased risk during training (so called "instructional issues"), which is reflected in the high proportion of dual seat gliders in the accident figures.[12] Most gliding accidents occur during landing (61% in 1985) or takeoff (16%), although the latter is more likely to have a fatal outcome and accounted for nearly half the fatalities in 1977–1981.[13] Most landing accidents are survivable, probably because of the low landing speed combined with effective harness restraint, but leg and back injuries are common because there is no cushioning structure to protect these regions. There is no cause for complacency, and it is to be hoped that the association may yet consider some degree of formal aviation medicine training for its members, perhaps as a part of its recently introduced Flight Safety Regulations, while striving to maintain and improve safety standards: for example, most glider pilots do not wear protective helmets, although constraints of space make redesign of cockpits, or preferably helmets, a prerequisite of wider acceptance. Furthermore, stricter medical requirements, which at present consist only of a signed declaration of physical fitness, should be imposed, or perhaps the Civil Aviation Authority should reconsider whether to include all glider pilots in its medical licensing scheme, as is the case in Canada and elsewhere.

Hang gliders

Hang gliders were developed in the 1960s from the design of a NASA employee, Francis Rogallo. Since the 1970s hang gliding has become a growing and fashionable sport, but the limited manoeuvrability, susceptibility to sudden wind changes and lack of body protection for the pilot combine to make the activity relatively dangerous. In the United Kingdom, the sport is carefully controlled by the British Hang Gliding Association which lays down training requirements and recommends appropriate safety equipment[14] such as a protective helmet (which is mandatory for association members during training and when flying in competitions), a high quality harness, adequate clothing—in particular strong footwear—and a parachute. Although heavy, oxygen equipment is a requirement for high altitude hang gliding. In North America, however, where cross country hang gliding is often carried out at 4267 m (14 000 ft) or above, the cavalier attitude to such protection occasionally defies belief: ". . . at 18 500 ft . . . I was now on oxygen. I didn't have a mask, so I just stuck the tube in my mouth and this worked tolerably well."[15] A British hang gliding enthusiast, having attended an aviation medicine training course, displayed a more commendable attitude and even commented on the relevance of disorientation during hang gliding.[16] Most medical interest in this sport has, however, centred on the injuries sustained and suggestions for preventing or reducing them. During the second half of the 1970s, in the wake of an increasing number of serious accidents, hang gliding accidents in various parts of the world were analysed.[17-21] Of reported accidents—and at that time reporting was not mandatory in many countries (and often is still not)—4–10% were fatal. Most fatalities were caused by head injuries, although the frequency of these was relatively low, probably because of the widespread use of protective helmets. Most major injuries were fractures or fracture–dislocations of the arms (36%) or legs (43%), and most (82%) occurred during takeoff or landing. Human error was to blame in most cases, often as a result of inexperience leading to poor choice of takeoff or landing sites, poor landing technique, and incorrect assessment of wind conditions, altitude, and speed.[18-22] Nevertheless, experienced pilots were not exempt.[20,21] Recommendations regarding licensing, ground training, and the use of safety equipment[18,20] have largely been adopted by the association (as outlined above) and, although the sport remains dangerous (there were two fatal hang gliding accidents in the United Kingdom in 1990 (but six in 1987)),[11] it is now possibly no more so than many other activities such as motor cycling, skiing, rock climbing, and horse riding.

Microlight aircraft

Microlight aircraft are the most recent entrants to sport flying and may best be described as powered hang gliders. These small lightweight machines can cruise at 112 kph (70 mph) and fly to altitudes above 4877 m (16 000 ft); the implications of this type of performance for aviation medicine are obvious. Perhaps at least partly as a result of public concern over hang gliding accidents and the increasing number of fatal microlight accidents, the Civil Aviation Authority has since September 1982 required microlights to be registered and their pilots to hold either a valid pilot's licence or to be flying under the supervision of a qualified flying instructor. Pilots must also hold a medical certificate, to which the usual disqualifying conditions apply. Whether such statutory requirements will reduce the morbidity and mortality rates of this pastime remains to be seen, but there were only three fatal microlight accidents in the United Kingdom in 1990, although there were seven in 1989.[11]

Helicopters

Helicopters first flew in the minds of men, and then as toys, in ancient China and medieval Europe. The first human-carrying, rotary wing flight occurred in 1907, when Paul Cornu—yet another Frenchman—flew at a height of a few feet for a few seconds, but it was not until 1938 that the first fully controlled helicopter flights were carried out. Since then there has been, and still is, an enormous expansion in the development, numbers, and use of rotary wing aircraft throughout the world. In terms of capability and adaptability, helicopters have become the aerial workhorses of this century. Quite apart from many military applications, helicopters are used in such varied civilian activities as commercial and executive transport, oil rig support and pipeline inspection, agricultural crop spraying, and emergency services. Despite this ubiquity helicopters have tended to be the cinderellas of aviation medicine. A consideration of the medical aspects of helicopter operations paints a fairly dismal picture with very few bright patches, but there are indications that this attitude is changing.

All the traditional aspects of aviation medicine are relevant to rotary wing flying, but the problems are compounded by movement in a third dimension. Furthermore, helicopters lack the static stability and control damping characteristic of fixed wing aircraft and are inherently more difficult to learn to control.

Comfort and thermal comfort

Flying a helicopter may be uncomfortable and very tiring, especially if no stability augmentation system is fitted. Physical discomfort is largely a result of vibration and more particularly of the operating position needed to fly the craft; both hands are occupied continuously, and because of the location of the control levers the pilot has to lean forward with little support for the upper half of the body. The discomfort to the back muscles is often compounded by poor seat design in relation to the flying controls. Frequently inadequate cushioning causes pelvic rotation and loss of lumbar lordosis, so that postural backache is a common complaint; this is often aggravated by the need to wear heavy and bulky protective clothing. The incidence of backache may, however, be minimised by preventing pelvic tilt through proper design of the seat cushion and by providing an adjustable lumbar support pad;[23] newer helicopters such as the Blackhawk are much better in this respect.

Thermal discomfort may cause further stress, particularly in military helicopters. Worldwide operations expose aircrew to extremes of temperature, and designers of military helicopters have usually not regarded cabin conditioning as a high priority. Thus even in a European summer the "greenhouse" effect of the cockpit transparency may produce cabin temperatures of over 40 °C during standby,[24] while in arctic conditions the lack of efficient cabin heating means that the pilot has to wear bulky clothing, which may impair precise operation of the aircraft.

For civilian operators, such as those supporting the North Sea oil industry, different constraints apply. Here the need is for clothing that is effective after ditching in seas at temperatures of

5–12 °C or below but ideally that does not have to be worn continuously in a heated cabin. The heat load of military type immersion suits was considered unacceptable for civilian flying, but new materials with enhanced ventile properties have improved this; both British Airways and Bristows Helicopters now require their helicopter crews to wear immersion suits when operating over the North Sea. Passengers on these services are also often required by their companies to wear protective clothing but the search continues for appropriate garments which can be put on quickly and worn continuously. Such clothing must be acceptable to the wearer, durable, and provide protection against drowning, hypothermia, and fire.[25]

Disorientation

Helicopter pilots and pilots of fixed wing aircraft are subject to the same types of disorientation (see chapter 7) and for both the "leans" is the most common problem: it has been reported by 96% and 91% respectively of those Royal Navy and United States Navy helicopter pilots questioned.[26,27] Head movements while in a bank or turn (51%), transition from instrument flight rules to visual flight rules and vice versa (42%), and misperception of the horizon because of a sloping cloudbank (46%) are also common problems during helicopter flying.[26] Similar figures for such events have been reported for land based military helicopter operations.[28]

Some phenomena are peculiar to rotary wing flying and are most liable to occur at low altitudes and at slow speeds or in a hover, with consequently very little time to correct mistakes. A helicopter is not only capable of conventional pitch, roll, and yaw movements but is also, in a controlled hover, susceptible to linear accelerations along these three axes. A pilot in the hover experiences a mixture of vestibular and proprioceptive stimuli which may be more difficult to interpret than those experienced in fixed wing aircraft. In general, forward acceleration is less disorienting than backward, lateral, or vertical acceleration.[27] There seems to be a particular vestibular insensitivity to vertical acceleration, so the hover is a time of increased risk. In the Royal Navy survey, disorientation frequently occurred in low hover under various conditions: over water by night in 29%, by day in 16%, under instrument flight rules in dust, snow, rain, or over water in 12%, and over land in 3%.[26] At night or in heavy snow ("whiteout") the loss of visual cues (a problem made worse by the restriction of the visual fields which occurs if night vision goggles are being worn) combined with relatively few vestibular inputs predisposes to disorientation; by day an illusory perception of motion may be generated by the movement of external visual cues. For example, when hovering over water or long grass a pilot may experience a false sensation of forward movement as the rotor downwash creates a rearward moving wave pattern. Similarly, a false sensation of upward motion may be generated by the downward movement of snow, rain, or entrained water through the rotor disc.[29] Should disorientation develop in this way, the situation is often helped by increasing forward airspeed and by flying straight and level. Other problems include annoyance, confusion, and occasional epileptiform episodes caused by flicker from the rotor blades or from lights seen through the rotor disc—"flicker vertigo"[28]—and the breakoff phenomenon[30] (see chapter 7).

Several factors, both specific to the aircraft and in general, compound the risk to the pilot of becoming disoriented. In a helicopter, internal reflections on the cockpit transparency, the reflection of anticollision lights on cloud or fog, and most importantly the inability to read instruments because of vibration are the most frequent predisposing factors. Fatigue, discomfort, upper respiratory tract infection, self medication, lack of recent instrument flying, insufficient flight planning, and inexperience all add to the risk.[26,27]

Fortunately, most episodes of disorientation do not progress to accidents. Nevertheless, in military flying 3–4% of helicopter accidents in the United States Army[31] and 15% in the British army[32] were considered to have disorientation as the major cause and in both cases accounted for nearly one-third of all fatalities. Improvements in these figures, which have remained remarkably constant over recent years,[29] will depend on modified and vibration damped instrumentation, additional cockpit aids (such as cathode ray tube displays and simple, peripheral vision horizon devices), and realistic training schemes both in the air and on the ground.[26,27,32,33]

Vision

A true visual horizon is essential for maintaining a selected attitude in helicopters because of their inherent instability. Most helicopter flying is, therefore, carried out while the pilot can see the ground or the surface of the sea, although flight in bad weather or at night is undertaken using instruments or night vision goggles respectively. Landing, however, still requires good external visual cues. These cues are modified in flight by many factors (see chapter 7) including motion perspective—that is, the apparent flow of stationary objects, or the surface, relative to the pilot's eyes.[34] This apparent flow indicates to the pilot the velocity, direction of movement, and approach path of the aircraft with respect to other objects or surfaces, and is common to fixed wing and rotary wing flying until the latter involves hovering.

In helicopters, flow perspective can be appreciated in all three planes of movement and provides one of the more important cues for aircraft control. In some circumstances, however, problems may arise. In the hover motion perspective, combined with absence of texture, produces the illusions of movement and consequent disorientation described above. Similar visual illusions of motion can occur at night when ground lights are reflected in cockpit transparencies, and this effect is a cause of serious incidents during flight.[35]

Approach and landing are also influenced visually by other distance cues such as size, density, and parallax. So called "pinnacle approaches"—landing on small, projecting, sites such as mountain tops or oil rig platforms—are particularly likely to produce problems of this sort. For this reason suitably textured landing sites in daylight—preferably with some indication of scale—and appropriately dispersed landing light patterns at night are needed. The hazard presented by wires is another visual problem. The distance at which they are detected depends on their size, the background against which they are located, and the ambient visual conditions. Wirestrikes are a major cause of military and agricultural helicopter accidents (for example the United States Army suffered 167 wirestrike accidents which caused 60 injuries and 34 fatalities during the period 1974–1981[36]), and active research into providing warning systems to help pilot visual acuity is being undertaken. Many helicopters are now fitted with wire cutting devices.

Noise and communication

Many helicopters are very noisy indeed; internal noise levels above 100 dB may occur in military helicopters during flight.[37] Together with discomfort, noise is the major complaint of helicopter occupants. Such high noise levels reduce communication efficiency, increase workload and fatigue, and if sufficiently high and prolonged can produce temporary and even permanent hearing loss: among United States Army helicopter pilots 30–40% develop high frequency sensorineural hearing loss to a degree which requires a waiver to allow continued flying. Predictably the noise in helicopters derives from the transmission, which produces a broad band spectrum of noise with additional large spikes produced by the main and tail rotor blades. The gearbox contributes to the broad band noise and produces smaller spikes. Aerodynamic noise from poorly streamlined surfaces adds to the load, particularly because many helicopters are inadequately sealed and are often flown with the windows and doors open or removed.

Communication input takes place for about 40% of the time during an average flight and is a major part of the total noise dose.[38] In addition, audio signals may be distorted during reception and amplification before they reach the recipient, and are further degraded by extraneous cabin noise. Cabin noise should therefore be reduced to improve the signal-to-noise ratio and decrease the total noise dose; ideally, speech signals should also be reduced both in magnitude and quantity.

The problems of noise reduction and improvement in communication should be tackled during the design stage of a helicopter's development, for example by carefully siting engines and gearboxes, isolating the cabin from noise and vibration sources as far as possible, and selecting a communication system with frequencies that do not conflict with noise peaks of other equipment. Because many helicopters have not been designed with such forethought, secondary measures need to be adopted to counter the problems. A modern protective helmet or headset with efficient noise dampening properties helps reduce the effects of cabin noise, but the low frequencies commonly encountered in helicopters are more difficult to attenuate, and audio signals at such frequencies may either be lost or need to be so high as to be hazardous themselves. The size of the audio workload may be a problem with the operator having to monitor several radio frequencies simultaneously. A wide range of possible signals makes learning, recognition, and response in emergencies more difficult. When these problems are added to the already sizeable normal audio input, the capacity of the operator may easily be exceeded. Verbal warning systems are now being considered, as load sharing in multicrew helicopters can provide only a partial solution. The amount of noise impinging on the ears is also reduced by effective noise cancelling microphones and voice operated switches.

Vibration

Vibration—defined as any sustained, mechanical, oscillatory disturbance perceived by senses other than hearing[39]—may be a source of annoyance and even a hazard during helicopter operations. Helicopters vibrate in all major axes and at frequencies related both to rotor speeds and to flight conditions, while further vibrations are produced by the engines, gearboxes and tail rotors. The effect of these vibrations, usually of low frequency (1–50 Hz) but sometimes of considerable energy, is exacerbated in certain flight conditions. The greatest body resonance occurs at 4–5 Hz and is related to the dynamics of the thorax and abdomen, but energy at these frequencies is usually low. The effect on visual performance is of greater concern: interpretation of instruments, target tracking through sights, and even the view of the outside world may be impaired if vibration levels are excessive. Vibration may also be a factor in the development of backache in helicopter crews.[40] The effects of vibration depend not only on body build, weight, and posture but also on the direction, area, intensity, and duration of application. Such equipment as seat cushions and harnesses also influence its effects.

Vibration in helicopters may be reduced externally by careful design of engines and rotors, and internally by instruments which are spring mounted or damped in some other way. Transmission of vibration to the occupants should be minimised as far as possible. A seat separated mechanically from the airframe by springs is one effective method of achieving this, especially when used with a five-point harness and a cushion made of energy absorbing material.[41]

Fatigue

Fatigue may be taken to denote those changes in physiology, decrease in work output (either in quantity or in quality), and characteristic subjective feelings of tiredness or disinclination to work which are associated with a continuous activity. It affects the efficiency and accuracy of aircraft operations and is an important cause of helicopter accidents. Of 120 peacetime military helicopter accidents, fatigue was a major contributory cause in 15%,[42] while in a United States Army series covering 7 years and 1270 accidents[43] fatigue related accidents (4% of the total) were four times more common in helicopters than in fixed wing aircraft. In a detailed analysis of the factors believed to promote fatigue, three main areas were important: long term workload, duty day workload, and short term workload.[42] When *long term workload* is assessed, scheduling of work and rest cycles, social and emotional factors, and morale have to be considered. *Duty day workload* covers the duration of work and rest periods throughout a given period of duty, while immediate or *short term workload* involves such factors as vibration, aircraft noise, limited visibility, instrument flying, and seat comfort.

Acute fatigue is produced by excessive mental or physical activity or both, and is often related to specific work situations: it is usually relieved by a period of sleep or rest. Operationally, the acutely fatigued pilot shows a fall in the level of skill while accepting, without being aware of it, a lower standard of accuracy and performance. Coning of attention is also likely. *Chronic fatigue* develops if the acute phase is not alleviated. Chronic fatigue does not respond to simple rest or a period of sleep, and those afflicted often have feelings of intense fatigue even before beginning work. In addition to the features of acute fatigue there is a decline in motivation, morale, and the quality of decision making.

Despite these apparently clear cut descriptions, a high index of suspicion is needed to detect victims of fatigue. Clinical features may include irritability with associated anxiety and depression, insomnia, social and vocational withdrawal, and excessive use of tobacco, drugs, or alcohol. There may also be a pronounced decline in attention span, short term memory, and cooperation, while physically there may be a loss of appetite, weight, and libido, and gastrointestinal problems may arise. The differential diagnoses include neurosis and physical disease, but there are no confirmatory behavioural or biochemical tests.

The causal factors indicate the preventive measures that should be considered: most—such as physical fitness, adequate recreational facilities, and sleep—are obvious. Less obvious, perhaps, is the need to adhere to the concept of a duty day in which time on duty, whether flying or not, is strictly regulated. In addition, the scope of expected tasks should be carefully and fully briefed, although this may be difficult to achieve without restricting the versatility of the helicopter. In the long term, the effects of many of the adverse immediate workload factors could be minimised by careful instrument and cockpit layout, more efficient control of the environment, and consideration of the ergonomics of seat and harness design.[44] Where prevention fails, however, the treatment is complete rest.

Impact protection and restraint

Accidents to helicopters may be divided into those that follow autorotation or forced landings and so are "controlled", and those that are uncontrolled such as wirestrikes or catastrophic impacts. (Autorotation is "the process of producing lift with freely rotating aerofoils by means of the aerodynamic forces resulting from an upward flow of air",[45] that is, non-powered flight.) Generally uncontrolled accidents are not survivable, but "controlled" accidents, which comprise over 90% of the total,[46] potentially are so. Such potentially survivable accidents in military helicopters account for 30–40% of occupant fatalities, with fire as the single largest cause of death.[46,47] A study of civilian helicopter accidents in the United States over 12 years also showed that 10% of 280 deaths resulted from fire after impact.[48] A fuel fire after a helicopter crash reaches its maximum intensity—with temperatures of 1093–1149 °C—just 15–20 s after a single point ignition such as might occur after a controlled impact.[49] Thus, if the occupants of a helicopter in this sort of accident are prevented from escaping rapidly from the craft and a fire develops they have little chance of survival. The safety aspects of helicopter crashworthiness are therefore largely concerned with ensuring that even mildly incapacitating injuries do not occur, and that victims are able to escape. Recognised shortcomings in the design of most modern helicopters are common to both civilian and military aircraft and include problems of rollover, intrusion of structures into the cockpit, seat failure, lack of restraint, and restraint failure.

Rollover, with subsequent disintegration of the cabin, may occur if on vertical impact the main rotors flex downwards and sever the tail boom. Similarly, a hard landing with a horizontal component may cause earth scooping and somersaulting of the fuselage. Subsequent intrusion into the cockpit by the engines, rotor blades, or cabin walls has a predictable outcome. The effects of equipment displacement in the passenger compartment may be partly reduced by the "delethalisation" of sharp edges and protuberances, and may be further minimised by the use of an appropriate protective helmet.

Helicopter crew seats frequently do not match the impact

tolerance of their occupants: on vertical impact the seats often collapse completely or break away from their mounts without appreciably reducing the applied force. Alternatively, the cushion alone may compress rapidly but without absorbing energy, so creating a dynamic overshoot and subjecting the victim to an amplified force as he or she is decelerated on contact with the underlying seat structure. Both mechanisms have resulted in serious injuries or death.[48] The problem is even worse for passengers: their seats are often constructed of tubular steel and are usually inadequately mounted. The advent of energy absorbing devices, which allow controlled displacement, has enabled improved seating to be introduced in United States military helicopters in accordance with the United States Army's Crash Survival Design Guide.[50] This extensive guide is an evolving document and design standards must, because the mechanism of crashes vary, be tailored to each specific aircraft so that costs can be reduced at the same time as crash protection is increased.[51] Although the United Kingdom has no equivalent document, the measures suggested in the American publication are generally accepted and implemented as far as possible.[52]

In many civilian helicopters crew members are restrained solely by a lap strap, which produces the inherent danger of jack-knifing. Even a four-point harness, with double lap and shoulder straps, does not prevent submarining. To overcome these risks a five-point harness, which includes a "negative G" strap, is now fitted to most military helicopters in the United Kingdom and has the additional advantages of preventing upward movement of the harness during vertical vibration in flight and of positioning the quick release fitting correctly.[41] Passengers are usually restrained by a simple lap strap, but to prevent jack-knifing and provide some protection against impact in the longitudinal axis of the aircraft a diagonal strap which passes over the leading shoulder when sitting sideways should also be provided at the very least. The geometry of harnesses is often poor, however, and better restraint is achieved in practice by the adoption of the crash posture, which prevents flail injuries and reduces the impact load on the spine. Harnesses for those required to move about the cabin must also be considered.

Although retrospective improvements to seats and restraint systems can only be for the good, safety features should be incorporated during the design stage to improve crashworthiness and to prevent accidents in the first place. It should be possible to overcome many of the problems known to cause accidents. Twin engines could be provided with duplicated, fracture resistant pipework and self sealing, fire resistant fuel systems: there have been no fire fatalities in survivable United States Army helicopter accidents since crashworthy fuel systems were introduced. Energy absorbing material could be used for seats and landing gear, while the crew/passenger compartments could be reinforced to prevent intrusion. Warning systems for detecting cables during flight exist, as do mechanisms for cutting them if hit. Theoretically, even automatic escape in flight is possible using individual rocket ejection/extraction or a passenger capsule escape facility.[53] Increased development and production costs, and reduced payload capacity, are usually given as reasons for failing to embody safety features, but a study of the cost effectiveness of many such measures incorporated in the Sikorsky UH-60A (Blackhawk) helicopter[54] has shown that a balanced solution in terms of cost, weight, and improved safety—as indicated by lives and aircraft saved—is certainly possible.[55]

Supersonic transport aircraft

In 1963, at an early stage in the Concorde project, the Anglo-French Concorde Aeromedical Group was formed to consider the aeromedical problems presented by such an advanced aircraft. The most important of these problems are created by Concorde's high cruising altitude of 18 288 m (60 000 ft).

Loss of cabin pressure

Sudden decompression to altitudes exceeding 15 850 m (52 000 ft) results in unconsciousness within 15 s of exposure whether air or pure oxygen is breathed.[56] Oxygen provides adequate protection for healthy subjects to an altitude of 12 192 m (40 000 ft); for passengers such a supply is available from drop down emergency sets. Protection above this altitude is adequate only if the oxygen is supplied under pressure so that an alveolar oxygen tension greater than 7·98 kPa (60 mmHg) is maintained.[56] The flight crew of Concorde is therefore provided with a supply of oxygen delivered at a mask pressure not exceeding 3·99 kPa (30 mmHg). The mask has been specially designed to meet

183

the licensing authorities' requirement that it can be put on within 5 s, which ensures that under the worst possible conditions of decompression the crew is sufficiently protected to start an emergency descent.

The main protection to Concorde's occupants is, however, derived from its deliberately "over engineered" design. The engineering safeguards include a considerable reserve capacity to supply air to the cabin, and the use of small windows (less than 15·2 cm diameter). Thus, if a window is lost at 19 812 m (65 000 ft) the maximum cabin altitude would reach only 10 973 m (36 000 ft) provided that an emergency descent was started within 30 s, and cabin altitude would be restored to about 4572 m (15 000 ft) within 6·5 min. The overall design is such that the cabin altitude will exceed 7620 m (25 000 ft) only after an extremely remote failure (less than one in 10^7 flying hours).[57] No decompression incidents have yet been reported during Concorde's commercial service.

Cosmic (ionising) radiation

We are all exposed to two types of extraterrestrial radiation. *Galactic radiation* originates from outside the solar system to produce a steady, reasonably predictable, low intensity flux of high energy particles.[58] The earth's magnetic field deflects the particles to give considerable protection in equatorial regions, but this effect declines to zero as the polar regions are approached, so that radiation at the poles is about twice that at the equator. Further protection is also afforded by the solar interplanetary magnetic field, and by the stratospheric absorption of low energy particles. The importance of this absorptive process is that the background radiation dose increases with altitude so that at its cruising altitude (18 288 m, 60 000 ft) Concorde is exposed to a galactic radiation dose of about twice that to which subsonic long haul aircraft are exposed at their cruising altitude of about 12 190 m (40 000 ft). Total supersonic and subsonic exposure levels will, however, be very similar because for equivalent routes the former's flight time is about half that of the latter.

The second type of radiation is *solar radiation*, the particles being released from the sun by solar flares. This radiation is of lower energy than galactic radiation, but its production, while unpredictable, may be intense.[58]

In 1991, in the light of new evidence based on interpolation of data from Japanese victims which suggested that previous recommendations were too optimistic, the International Commission on Radiation Protection recommended new limits for exposure to ionising radiation for workers and members of the public.[59] The recommended whole body dose for the former is now 20 mSv per year (previously 50), and is 1 mSv per year for the latter (previously 5). Additionally, the maximum recommended total exposure to the abdomen during pregnancy is 2 mSv.

The potential risk of exposure to ionising radiation for the occupants of Concorde has always been recognised but, because adequate physical shielding would impose uneconomic weight penalties on the aircraft, the radiation dose is monitored by a detector mounted near the top of the hull with its output displayed on the flight deck. The detector responds to charged particles, γ radiation and neutrons, and signal processing produces a single dose equivalent rate in $mrem\,h^{-1}$. The crew is alerted (amber warning) if the dose rate exceeds $10\,mrem\,h^{-1}$ ($0.1\,mSv\,h^{-1}$), while descent is mandatory if checks confirm an indicated dose rate in excess of $50\,mrem\,h^{-1}$ ($0.5\,mSv\,h^{-1}$): a red warning. During the past 20 years, British Airways and Air France Concorde aircraft have flown over 80 000 sectors and not once has a descent been initiated because of high radiation levels, even during times of high solar activity:[60] indeed, the average dose rate for the 3 years 1988–1990, during which Concordes made 6111 flights and flew for over 18 000 hours, was just $0.011\,mSv\,h^{-1}$. This was also the average dose rate for Concorde operations for the period 1976–1983.[61]

When these figures are applied to Concorde aircrew, an average annual dose of 3–4 mSv is derived, with a maximum of twice this; for cabin crew the average dose is 2–3 mSv with a maximum of 4–5 mSv. Clearly, therefore, ionising radiation should not be regarded as a risk for this population.[60]

Concern has also been expressed about the radiation risk to other aircrew, and specifically to those involved with the increasingly common long haul (>6 hours) and ultralong haul (>16 hours) operations. Many of these flights are transpolar, and consequently have the potential for high radiation exposure, but the computed figures reveal that even in the unrealistic case of continuous flying on polar routes, the maximum dose would again be a safe 6 mSv per year.

For casual passengers, too, the new recommendations pose little problem: the annual limit of 1 mSv equates to about 100 hours of Concorde or subsonic transpolar flying or 200 hours of subsonic transequatorial flying. The limit could, however, be easily exceeded by a business traveller. The Commission has taken a pragmatic approach to this and supports the notion that such flying is essentially occupational, and so can be governed by the higher limit. Under these guidelines a business traveller could cross the Atlantic every day of the year with impunity.

Pregnant aircrew and pregnant business travellers could be expected to exceed the recommended gestational dose after about 200 hours flying time, but it is likely that flying during pregnancy will be curtailed for other reasons long before this happens.

Ozone

Ozone (O_3) is a strong oxidising agent produced by the action of ultraviolet light on oxygen (O_2). At ground level its concentration is about 0·03 parts per million by volume (ppmv), but this increases rapidly above 12 192 m (40 000 ft) to reach a maximum of about 10 ppmv at 30 480 m (100 000 ft). At Concorde's normal cruising altitude the ozone concentration is about 4 ppmv, but this depends on latitude and season.[62]

The toxic effects of ozone in humans are predominantly respiratory. Acute exposure for 2 hours to low concentrations of 0·6–0·8 ppm considerably reduces the diffusing capacity for carbon monoxide, probably by causing alveolar oedema, and slightly reduces vital capacity and forced expiratory volume.[63] In a long term study of two groups exposed for 3 hours a day to 0·2 or 0·5 ppm no reduction in forced vital capacity or forced expiratory volume was observed during 12 weeks at the lower dose. Over the same period, however, the higher dose group showed a statistically significant fall in forced expiratory volume but no change in forced vital capacity, indicating a degree of bronchiolar obstruction.[64] The forced expiratory volume had returned to normal when remeasured 6 weeks after exposure ceased. Ozone also impairs night vision in humans,[65] and in human cell cultures can induce chromatid breakages that are apparently identical to those produced by X-rays.[66] This radiomimetic action of ozone has also been suggested by studies in rabbits and mice.[67] Under simulated flight conditions, ozone produces eye discomfort, headache, and nasal and throat irritation.[68]

Fortunately, ozone is thermally unstable and its decomposition to oxygen is complete at 400 °C, the temperature reached by Concorde's air conditioning compressor circuit during climb and cruising. During these phases of flight the cabin concentration of ozone may be expected to remain below 0·1 ppmv: the concentration set as a maximum for industrial workers exposed to ozone for a 5-day, 40-hour week. On descent, compressor temperature falls to about 300 °C, giving an ozone dissociation rate of about 90%, and the maximum exposure is then likely to be 0·25 ppmv for 3 min. Actual measurements in Concorde[69] have indicated that at 15 240 m (50 000 ft) ozone could not be detected in the cabin despite an external ozone concentration of 1·5 ppm. On descent maximum values were 0·16 ppm, but a concentration of 0·1 ppm was exceeded for only 4 min.[69] Such figures compare favourably with values in subsonic aircraft of 20–30 years ago,[62,64] but more recent studies have demonstrated ozone concentrations in excess of the exposure standards.[70] Because of this, it is likely that future aircraft, whether supersonic or subsonic, will be fitted with catalytic converters.

Kinetic heating

At Mach 2 some external aircraft structures may reach temperatures of 150 °C.[57] To prevent unacceptable increases in its temperature the cabin is double walled, and air is passed between the walls at high flows. Because the dynamic air is very hot at Mach 2, however, it is first cooled by conventional heat exchangers and cold compressors and also by heat exchange with the aircraft's fuel. The temperature of the air entering the cabin is then closely controlled to ensure a steady cabin temperature of 24 °C (range 22–27 °C).

Noise

The noise levels inside Concorde are similar to those in subsonic aircraft because of Concorde's extensive soundproofing. The major source of noise is external, although at subsonic speeds Concorde's noise levels compare favourably with those of conventional jet aircraft such as the DC8: both produce noise levels of about 115 dB on takeoff and approach.[57] The advent of quieter, new generation, subsonic jets—for example, the Airbus, which has an approach noise level of 102 dB—means that Concorde will be one of the noisier aircraft flying in the early 1990s.

Sonic boom and "super boom"[71] have caused a great deal of discussion and annoyance, but their medical effects have been poorly defined. At present, Concorde does not fly supersonic over land, but a supersonic corridor was provided over the middle east when British Airways operated a supersonic service to Bahrain.

1 Taylor JWR, Munson K, eds. *History of aviation.* London: New English Library, 1975: 506.
2 Engle E, Lott AS. *Man in flight—biomedical achievements in aerospace.* Maryland: Leeward Publications, 1979: 1–29.
3 Ernsting J. Prevention of hypoxia—acceptable compromises. *Aviat Space Environ Med* 1978; **49:** 495–502.
4 Ross MD. We saw the world from the edge of space. *National Geographic* 1961; **120:** 670–85.
5 Axelsson R, Danewid R, Petersson Å, eds. *The world soaring directory.* Skövde, Sweden: Swedish Gliding Journal, 1989.
6 Scull B. Workload management and flying to the limits. *Sailplane and Gliding* 1982; **Feb/March:** 19.
7 Anonymous. Disorientation in flight. *Sailplane and Gliding* 1980; **Feb/March:** 18–19.
8 Murray Wilson A. Oxygen and altitude for glider pilots. *Sailplane and Gliding* 1986; **June/July:** 122–3.
9 British Gliding Association. *Laws and rules for glider pilots,* 11th edn. Leicester: British Gliding Association, 1992: 42–4.
10 New Products—Electronic Delivery System. *Soaring* 1993; **57:** 48.
11 Civil Aviation Authority. *Reportable accidents to UK registered aircraft, and to foreign registered aircraft in UK airspace, 1990.* London: Civil Aviation Authority, 1992. (CAP 600:x).
12 British Gliding Association. *Accidents to gliders—1992.* Leicester: British Gliding Association, 1993.
13 British Gliding Association. *Accidents to gliders—1977–1981.* Leicester: British Gliding Association.
14 Welsh A, ed. *The BHGA pilot handbook.* Taunton: British Hang Glider Association, 1979.
15 Pollard M. Rendezvous with a glider. *Wings!* 1982; **March:** 20–2.
16 Hudson JA. Twenty-five thousand feet gentlemen—uncouple your oxygen. *Wings!* 1981; **June:** 14–15.
17 Krissoff WB, Eiseman B. Injuries associated with hang-gliding. *JAMA* 1975; **233:** 158–60.
18 Yuill GM. Icarus's syndrome: new hazards in flight. *BMJ* 1977; **i:** 823–5.
19 Tongue JR. Hang-gliding injuries in California. *J Trauma* 1977; **17:** 898–902.
20 Margreiter R, Lugger L-J. Hang-gliding accidents. *BMJ* 1978; **i:** 400–2.
21 Anonymous. Hang-gliding accidents (editorial). *NZ Med J* 1979; **89:** 481–2.
22 Anonymous. Hazards of hang-gliding (editorial). *BMJ* 1978; **i:** 388.
23 Steele-Perkins AP. The evolution of the helicopter seat-pan mounted personal survival pack. In: Auffret R, ed. *Aircrew safety and survivability.* Neuilly-sur-Seine, France: NATO Advisory Group for Aerospace Research and Development, 1980; A16.1–A16.3. (AGARD Conference Proceedings No 286.)
24 Harrison MH, Higenbottam C. Heat stress in an aircraft cockpit during ground standby. *Aviat Space Environ Med* 1977; **48:** 519–23.
25 Leese WLB, Norman JN. Helicopter passenger survival suit standards in the UK offshore oil industry. *Aviat Space Environ Med* 1979; **50:** 110–14.
26 Steele-Perkins AP, Evans DA. Disorientation in Royal Naval helicopter pilots. In: Knapp SC, ed. *Operational helicopter aviation medicine.* Neuilly-sur-Seine, France: NATO Advisory Group for Aerospace Research and Development, 1978; 48.1–48.5. (AGARD Conference Proceedings No 255.)
27 Tormes FR, Guedry FE. *Disorientation phenomena in naval helicopter pilots.* Pensacola, FL: Naval Aerospace Research Laboratory 1974; NAMRL-1205.
28 Clarke B. Pilot reports of disorientation across 14 years of flight. *Aerospace Med* 1971; **42:** 708–12.
29 Turner JCD. Medical aspects of special types of flight—helicopters. In: Ernsting J, King PF, eds. *Aviation medicine,* 2nd edn. London: Butterworths, 1988: 475.
30 Benson AJ. Spatial disorientation and the "break-off" phenomenon. *Aerospace Med* 1973; **44:** 944–52.
31 Ogden FW, Jones QW, Chappell HR. Disorientation experiences of army helicopter pilots. *Aerospace Med* 1966; **37:** 140–3.

32 Edgington K, Box CJ. Disorientation in army helicopter operations. *J Soc Occup Med* 1982; **32:** 128–35.

33 Benson AJ, Burchard E. *Spatial disorientation in flight—a handbook for aircrew.* Neuilly-sur-Seine, France: NATO Advisory Group for Aerospace Research and Development, 1973. (AGARDograph No 170.)

34 Mackie WAN. Operation of helicopters—some visual problems. In: Fryer DI, ed. *Aeromedical aspects of helicopter operations in the tactical situation.* Paris: NATO Advisory Group for Aerospace Research and Development, 1967: 157–63. (AGARD Conference Proceedings No 24.)

35 Eastwood HK, Berry CA. Disorientation in helicopter pilots. *Aerospace Med* 1960; **31:** 191–9.

36 Farr WD, Ruehle CJ, Posey DM, Wagner GN. Injury pattern analysis of helicopter wire strike accidents (− Gz load). *Aviat Space Environ Med* 1985; **56:** 1216–19.

37 Rood GM. *Measurement of cabin noise in Puma HC1 helicopters.* Farnborough: Royal Aircraft Establishment, 1976. (Technical Memorandum FS 97.)

38 Rood GM, Lovesay EJ. Some aspects of helicopter communications. In: Knapp SC, ed. *Operational helicopter aviation medicine.* Neuilly-sur-Seine, France: NATO Advisory Group for Aerospace Research and Development, 1978: 47.1–47.7. (AGARD Conference Proceedings No 255.)

39 Stott JRR. Vibration. In: Ernsting J, King PF, eds. *Aviation medicine*, 2nd edn. London: Butterworths, 1988: 185.

40 Delahaye RP, Auffret R, Merges PJ, Poirer JL, Vettes B. Backache in helicopters. In: Delahaye RP, Auffret R, eds. *Physiopathology and pathology of spinal injuries*, 2nd edn. Neuilly-sur-Seine, France: Advisory Group for Aerospace Research and Development, 1982: 226. (AGARDograph No 250.)

41 Reader DC. Some improvements to the UK helicopter cockpit. In: Knapp SC, ed. *Operational helicopter aviation medicine.* Neuilly-sur-Seine, France: NATO Advisory Group for Aerospace Research and Development, 1978: 60.1–60.3. (AGARD Conference Proceedings No 255.)

42 Perry IC, ed. *Helicopter aircrew fatigue.* Neuilly-sur-Seine, France: NATO Advisory Group for Aerospace Research and Development, 1974. (AGARD Advisory Report No 69.)

43 Krueger GP, Jones YF. US army aviation fatigue-related accidents, 1971–1977. In: Knapp SC, ed. *Operational helicopter aviation medicine.* Neuilly-sur-Seine, France: NATO Advisory Group for Aerospace Research and Development, 1978: 20.1–20.11. (AGARD Conference Proceedings No 255.)

44 Steele-Perkins AP. Ergonomics and the aviator. *J R Navy Med Serv* 1981; **67:** 147–9.

45 Fay J. *The helicopter—history, piloting and how it flies*, 3rd edn. London: David and Charles, 1976: 80.

46 Sand LD. Comparative injury patterns in US army helicopters. In: Knapp SC, ed. *Operational helicopter aviation medicine.* Neuilly-sur-Seine, France: NATO Advisory Group for Aerospace Research and Development, 1978: 54.1–54.7. (AGARD Conference Proceedings No 255.)

47 Haley JL. Analysis of US army helicopter accidents to define impact injury problems. In: *Linear acceleration of impact type.* Neuilly-sur-Seine, France: NATO Advisory Group for Aerospace Research and Development, 1971: 9.1–9.12. (AGARD Conference Proceedings No 88.)

48 Snyder RG. Occupant injury mechanisms in civil helicopter accidents. In: Knapp SC, ed. *Operational helicopter aviation medicine.* Neuilly-sur-Seine, France: NATO Advisory Group for Aerospace Research and Development, 1978: 53.1–53.14. (AGARD Conference Proceedings No 255.)

49 Knox FS, Wachtel TL, McCahan GR. Bioassay of thermal protection afforded by candidate flight suit fabrics. *Aviat Space Environ Med* 1979; **50:** 1023–30.

50 Zimmerman RE, Merritt NA. *Aircraft crash survival design guide. Volume 1—Design criteria and checklists.* Aviation Applied Technology Directorate, Fort Eustis, Virginia 1989. (USAAVSCOM Technical Report 89-D-22A.)

51 Shanahan DF, Shanahan MO. Kinematics of US army helicopter crashes: 1979–85. *Aviat Space Environ Med* 1989; **60:** 112–21.

52 Steele-Perkins AP. Recent improvements in crash restraint in UK helicopters. In: Haley JL, ed. *Impact injury caused by linear acceleration: mechanism, prevention and cost.* Neuilly-sur-Seine, France: NATO Advisory Group for Aerospace Research and Development, 1982: 27.1–27.9. (AGARD Conference Proceedings No 322.)

53 Reader DC. Helicopter escape and survivability. In: Nicholson AN, ed. *Fourth advanced operational aviation medicine course.* Neuilly-sur-Seine, France: NATO Advisory Group for Research and Development 1976: 67–8. (AGARD Report No 642.)

54 Carnell BL. Crash survivability of the UH-60A helicopter. In: Knapp SC, ed. *Operational helicopter aviation medicine.* Neuilly-sur-Seine, France: NATO Advisory Group for Research and Development 1978: 64.1–64.10. (AGARD Conference Proceedings No 255.)

55 Meller R. Emphasis on safety and survivability. *International Defence Review* 1978; **5:** 669–72.

56 Ernsting J. *Some effects of raised intrapulmonary pressure in man.* London: W and J Mackay, 1966: 1–20. (AGARDograph No 106.)

57 Preston FS. Medical aspects of supersonic travel. *Aviat Space Environ Med* 1975; **46:** 1074–8.

58 Wilson IJ. Radiation and supersonic flight. *Sci J* 1966; **66:** 31–7.

59 International Commission on Radiological Protection. Publication 60. *Ann ICRP* 1991; **21:** 1–3.

60 Davies DM. *Cosmic radiation in concorde operations and the impact of new ICRP recommendations on commercial aviation.* Radiation Protection Dosimetry 1993; **48:** 121–4.

61 Preston FS. Eight years experience of concorde operations: medical aspects. *J R Soc Med* 1985; **78:** 193.

62 Bischof W. Ozone measurements in jet airliner cabin air. *Water, Air and Soil Pollution* 1973; **2:** 3–14.

63 Young WA, Shaw DB, Bates DV. Effect of low concentrations of ozone on pulmonary function in man. *J Appl Physiol* 1964; **19:** 765–8.

64 Bennett G. Ozone contamination of high altitude aircraft cabins. *Aerospace Med* 1962; **33:** 969–73.

65 Lagerwerff JM. Prolonged ozone inhalation and its effects on visual parameters. *Aerospace Med* 1963; **34:** 479–86.

66 Fetner RH. Ozone-induced chromosome breakage in human cell cultures. *Nature* 1962; **194:** 793–4.

67 Brinkman R, Lamberts HB, Veninga TS. Radiomimetic toxicity of ozonised air. *Lancet* 1964; **i:** 133–6.

68 Lategola MT, Melton CE, Higgins EA. Effects of ozone on symptoms and cardiopulmonary function in a flight attendant surrogate population. *Aviat Space Environ Med* 1980; **51:** 237–46.

69 Leach JF, Sandals FJ. Measurement of ozone in Concorde cabin air. In: *Abstracts from the 26th international congress of aerospace medicine, London.* Basel: Geigy Pharmaceuticals, 1978: 12.

70 Nastrom GD, Holdeman JD, Perkins PJ. Measurements of cabin and ambient ozone on B747 airplanes. *J Aircraft* 1980; **17:** 246–9.

71 Andrew J. Subsonic and supersonic operations in the years ahead. *J R Aeronaut Soc* 1971; **75:** 269–79.

12
Manned spacecraft

We set sail on this new sea because there is new knowledge to be gained and new rights to be won, and they must be won and used for the progress of all people. For space science, like nuclear science and all technology, has no conscience of its own.

JF Kennedy (1917–1963)

Since Yuri Gagarin first orbited the earth on 12 April 1961 well over 200 human beings have journeyed into space, and it has become clear that microgravity (weightlessness) is the major physiological challenge in that environment. Before experiencing microgravity, however, a human must first be provided with a life support system and tolerate the increased accelerations imposed by the launch of the spacecraft.

Acceleration

A velocity of 8 km s^{-1} (28 800 kph, 17 900 mph) must be attained to enter earth orbit, while a velocity of 11·6 km s^{-1} (41 760 kph, 25 950 mph) is needed to escape the earth's gravitational field. Such velocities may be reached by an infinite number of combinations of acceleration and time, provided that their product is 828 G seconds for orbit or 1152 G seconds for escape. In practice the acceleration profile is limited by the design of rocket motors, which produce high thrust for only a relatively short period. The two-stage Gemini launch, for example, produced peak accelerations of 5·5 and 7·2 G.[1] During Apollo launches, accelerations were not much greater than 4 G, but re-entry from lunar missions produced levels of 6·7 G.[2] Soviet Soyuz spacecraft experience launch and re-entry accelerations of 3·0–4·0 G, but the earlier Vostok craft re-entered at an average maximum acceleration of 8·0–10·0 G.[3]

Because of hydrostatic circulatory effects, such levels of acceleration are poorly tolerated unless the body is exposed to them traversely ($+$ Gx) (see chapter 6). Thus astronauts adopt a reclined position during high accleration exposure. Human tolerance to $+$ Gx acceleration is limited by chest pain and an inability to breathe as a result of the increased effective weight of the chest wall. The latter is reflected by a reduced vital capacity: at $+$ 6 Gx, for example, vital capacity is halved.[4] Ventilation–perfusion inequalities are created and lung collapse may develop by the same mechanisms that produce such changes under $+$ Gz acceleration— except, of course, that the dependent lung is posterior rather than basal. Atelectasis does not, however, cause problems in space flight, but the right-to-left shunt will produce arterial oxygen desaturation, similar falls occurring whether air or an enriched oxygen supply is breathed.[5] Although these accelerations have proved to be tolerable, any reduction in their magnitude is desirable. The space shuttle's launch acceleration profile does not exceed 3·4 G, while its re-entry profile is a very sedate 1·2 Gz—but for 17 min (see below).[3]

Spacecraft environment

Cabin atmosphere

At 30 480 m (100 000 ft) the atmosphere pressure is a mere 1·09 kPa (8·2 mmHg), while at 300 km (186 miles) the value is about 1×10^{-11} times that at sea level. Air compression is, therefore, no longer a practical method of providing a cabin atmosphere. Instead, spacecraft use a pressurised sealed system which, for Soviet and American craft, is at sea level equivalent *pressure* for launch (101·3 kPa or 760 mmHg). The approach to atmospheric *composition* was, however, fundamentally different for the two programmes. The Soviets selected an atmosphere for launch and orbit similar in composition to that of air at sea level: 21% oxygen, 79% nitrogen.[6] Although physiologically ideal, this imposes weight and engineering penalties on the spacecraft, and because of the risk of decompression sickness cosmonauts are required to breathe 100% oxygen for up to an hour before undertaking extravehicular activity.

For the American Mercury and Gemini projects, the launch atmosphere was 100% oxygen, and this was maintained in orbit but at a reduced pressure of 34·5 kPa (259 mmHg). The single gas system had the advantage of simple engineering control, and because the gas was oxygen the risk of decompression sickness was minimised; although the transition from high launch to low orbital atmospheric pressures required a preoxygenation period before launch of 3 hours. There was, however, no subsequent requirement to preoxygenate before undertaking extravehicular activity.

Once in orbit, a sealed system requires only the addition of oxygen, to compensate for outboard leakage and respiratory consumption, and the removal of carbon dioxide.

The 100% oxygen system chosen by NASA was not, however, without hazard, particularly during launch. The fire risks of such an atmosphere had been suggested by work at the Royal Air Force Institute of Aviation Medicine[7] and were tragically confirmed by the fatal launch pad fire of Test Apollo 204 (later renamed Apollo 1 in honour of the crew) in January 1967. The cabin launch atmosphere for the Apollo launches was changed to 64% oxygen and 36% nitrogen at sea level pressure. After entry into orbit, the cabin pressure was again reduced to just over 34·5kPa (259 mmHg). Oxygen was used to purge nitrogen from the atmosphere through the valve used for discarding urine into space, and the oxygen content was gradually raised to over 90% by the third day of flight. Throughout the Apollo flights the partial pressure of oxygen was never less than its sea level equivalent.[2] Similar atmospheric conditions were provided for Skylab, except that orbital composition was 70% oxygen and 30% nitrogen.

The reduction in orbital oxygen content was also expected to have the benefit of preventing the decline in red cell mass—of up to 20%—which occurred in astronauts during flights before the Apollo missions.[2] This phenomenon was thought to be due to oxygen toxicity—a mechanism suggested by the haemolysis observed in mice exposed to hyperbaric oxygen.[8] No reduction in red cell mass occurred in the crews of Apollo 7 or 8 (the first manned Apollo missions), but it did recur in later Apollo flights and in all three Skylab missions. The loss of erythrocytes in Skylab crew members was associated with a lowered reticulocyte count, but isotopic measurements of red cell lifespan produced no evidence of haemolysis.[9] Similar changes have also been reported by the Soviets,[10] so that atmospheric pressure and composition are no longer considered to be prime aetiological factors; rather it is likely to be yet another direct consequence of microgravity (see below).

Portable life support system

During extravehicular activity, astronauts wear multilayered gas impermeable space suits which, for the Apollo/Skylab missions, were pressurised to a nominal 25·5 kPa (191 mmHg) with 100% oxygen supplied by a portable life support system backpack.[11] Although this pressure is the minimum that is physiologically acceptable, it allows more mobility than higher pressures which reduce suit flexibility. A ventilating circuit in the system ensures regular circulation of fresh oxygen after carbon dioxide and excess water have been removed. Although the oxygen is also cooled, this does not adequately control body temperature during some phases of activity when large heat loads are produced. For these occasions liquid refrigerant is cooled in the system and circulated through a network of plastic tubing in a "liquid conditioned garment" worn next to the skin. The portable life support system also includes an oxygen purge mechanism in case of loss of suit pressure, and sophisticated biotelemetry which permits ground based assessments of the astronaut's requirements for oxygen and cooling, as well as medical monitoring. Early Soviet spacesuits were pressurised to 40 kPa (300 mmHg) and were able to maintain adequate mobility, but recent Soviet extravehicular activities have been accomplished in lightweight suits pressurised to just 23·4 kPa (176 mmHg).[3]

For the space transportation system, the Shuttle, a sea level atmosphere is used for launch and for much of the mission in orbit. To reduce the time required for preoxygenation before extravehicular activity to an operationally acceptable period, however, the whole craft undergoes an intermediate depressurisation phase. Thus, for 12 hours before such an activity, cabin pressure is reduced to 70·3 kPa (527·3 mmHg) (that is, to 3048 m (10 000 ft) equivalent), and the oxygen concentration increased to about 27% (that is, to 1200 m (3900 ft) equivalent).[3] Those undertaking extravehicular activity then prebreathe 100% oxygen for 40 min before entering their spacesuits which are pressurised to 29·6 kPa (222·3 mmHg). Mobility is retained despite the increased pressure because the latest joint technology is used.

Waste collection

On American flights before Skylab, a plastic stoma bag and finger cot were used for defecation but predictably proved very unpopular with astronauts, not least because the process took up to 45 min to complete and, to preserve specimens, an antibacterial agent had to be added to the bag which was then kneaded to ensure thorough mixing! Urine was collected through colour coded condoms and rubber tubing. The Skylab astronauts had greater privacy in a purpose built toilet area which used electric air blowers to carry waste away from the user into collection bags. Faecal material was subsequently dried in a special processor and stowed for later analysis on earth. A similar system has been adopted for the shuttle, and the urine collecting device has been designed for use by men and women. Soviet waste disposal techniques have always been rather more refined, and even the earliest cosmonauts were spared the public contortions required by their American peers.[3]

Ionising radiation

Once beyond the protection of the earth's atmospheric blanket and its magnetic field, spacecraft and their occupants are exposed to the full power of the electromagnetic spectrum, and especially to ionising radiation. In space, to the hazards of galactic and solar radiation (see chapter 11) are added those of trapped radiation in the Van Allen belts and of energetic neutrons (unstable neutrons which, because of their propensity to collide with hydrogen nuclei to produce free radicals, are potentially very harmful to human tissues).[3] Not surprisingly, therefore, it had been predicted that radiation would be a serious medical threat to astronauts, particularly on lunar missions which necessitated passing through the Van Allen belts.[12]

The crews of Apollo 11, 12, and 13 reported seeing flashes of light which were later attributed to the penetration of the spacecraft by highly charged high Z energy particles of galactic radiation (Z is the atomic number of the element concerned) which produced visual sensations after interaction with the retina. Despite these observations the average radiation exposure on Apollo flights, as measured by passive dosimeters, was only 4 mGy (0·4 rad), with Apollo 14 receiving the highest dose of 11·4 mGy (1·14 rad) because of solar flare activity.[13] The highest mean cumulative doses recorded on American flights were during the 84-day Skylab 4 mission at 78·1 mGy (7·81 rad), but the exposure levels were well below permitted limits.[14] Soviet experience has been remarkably similar, with a mean daily skin dose of just 0·18 mGy (0·018 rad) during early Soyuz missions.

Thus, passive shielding by spacecraft walls and equipment has been effective so far, although careful flight scheduling has also played an important role. But with plans being considered for the long term occupation of stations in near and deep space, as well as for extended missions to other planets, other methods must be sought, such as pharmacological protection or active shielding by magnetic or electric field induction. For many, radiation is still regarded as "the primary source of hazard for orbital and interplanetary space flight".

Microgravity (weightlessness)

Space travellers are not actually exposed to zero gravity but to a microgravity of $1 \times 10^{-4} - 1 \times 10^{-5}$ G (during spacecraft manoeuvres this may increase to 1×10^{-3} G).[15] Although microgravity has its principal overt effects on the neurovestibular, cardiovascular, and musculoskeletal systems, no system is unaffected and important related changes are also seen in the endocrine system, the immune system and in haematology. Because observations have been possible on relatively few subjects (for whom countermeasures were widely utilised), additional data have been derived from ground simulations of prolonged microgravity, notably bed rest and water immersion. Clearly such simulations cannot duplicate weightless conditions because gravity is never completely eliminated; but recent evidence from cardiovascular studies on the Spacelab Life Sciences (SLS-1) shuttle mission in 1991 has helped to elucidate the bed rest model, and to shed more (and unexpected) light on possible underlying mechanisms.

Neurovestibular system

The most important early neurovestibular disturbance encountered in microgravity is space motion sickness, which forms a major part of the general space adaptation syndrome. By itself, microgravity does not induce space sickness; indeed, space sickness did not occur in American astronauts until the early Apollo missions. The 22 Mercury and Gemini astronauts were free of symptoms probably because their head movements were restricted by body restraint and lack of room.[16] The larger size of the Apollo spacecraft allowed more movement and, before the Apollo 10 mission, head movements were actually encouraged.[2] As a result, five of the six crewmen of Apollos 8 and 9 reported symptoms; and the overall incidence during the Apollo programme was 35%, while on Skylab it was 60%. During 24 missions of the space shuttle, the incidence was 67% for those on their first mission (24% being classed moderately severe, and 11% severe), falling to 26% for those on their second flight.[17] Similar problems have also been experienced throughout the Soviet spaceflight programme: the association between rapid head movements and malaise first being reported by Cosmonaut Titov, the second Soviet in space.[18] Thereafter the incidence was 50–60% during the early Vostok and Soyuz missions, and about 42% on the space stations Salyut 6 and 7.[17]

Space sickness produces symptoms similar to those of terrestrial motion sickness, and may be completely disabling. It usually occurs early in flight, but after 3 days most of those afflicted are able to move their heads without any discomfort: all except the scientist astronaut on Apollo 9 were free of symptoms after 6–7 days. This adaptation does not, however, afford protection against sea sickness on return to normal gravity. Furthermore, return is often associated with sensations of tumbling and vertigo similar to those experienced during microgravity. Physiologically, space sickness is probably due to absent or incorrect otolithic information which is at variance with normal semicircular canal cues[18] (see chapter 7). The possibility that the redistribution of body fluid during microgravity has a direct effect on the central nervous system is unlikely.[19]

Unfortunately, no laboratory test has yet been devised which accurately predicts an individual's susceptibility to space sickness, but Skylab experiments demonstrated that antiemetic drugs—for example, hyoscine—are partially effective in its prevention and treatment.[16] In the American programme a combination of hyoscine (scopolamine) and dexamphetamine ("Scop-Dex") has been found to be the most useful. Affected individuals also seek out other methods of ameliorating the illness such as wedging themselves in a corner to keep still, and trying to maintain an appropriately oriented visual scene: colleagues spinning in midair or floating past upside down do not help! The Soviets, with some success, have even employed a restraint system to keep the head still.

Other neurovestibular manifestations include postural illusions, dizziness, vertigo, and nystagmus. Such phenomena usually occur soon after entering microgravity and only last for a few hours; but they may recur throughout a mission and especially at times of increased motor or visual activity. Disorders of equilibrium and gross motor function, often manifest as an ataxia, have been observed in some but by no means all returning cosmonauts, especially after the longer Soviet Soyuz–Mir missions and particularly if assessments are made with the eyes shut. Recovery from this neurotaxic dysfunction may take weeks or months, and suggests that the importance of proprioceptive behaviour during and after flight may have been seriously underestimated.[20]

Cardiovascular system

Microgravity neutralises the hydrostatic pressure gradients in the circulation so that, in particular, venous pressures become uniform throughout the body. Immersion in water produces a central shift of about 700 ml of blood from the legs[21] but under weightless conditions the volume of blood and interstitial fluid displaced from the lower extremities is considerably greater— about 2 l.[22] This discrepancy cannot be completely explained by the total abolition of hydrostatic gradients and suggests that active as well as passive factors control the compliance of the interstitial space[15] and determine the distribution of fluid between the intravascular and extravascular compartments.

Changes in the cardiovascular system were first studied in the nine astronauts who took part in the three extended Skylab missions (28, 59, and 84 days). Fluid shifts were complete by the time measurements were first made on the third and fourth days of the flights. The shift is, however, probably accomplished within 24–48 h, because the astronauts noted sensations of fullness in the head and nasal stuffiness early in the missions.[23] Inflight photographs (both conventional and infrared) showed that all Skylab crew members had full, distended jugular and forehead veins, and the venous distension with its associated symptoms remained throughout flight.[2]

Until recently, it was thought that central volume expansion stimulated a diuresis via the Gauer–Henry reflex: suppression of arginine vasopressin (antidiuretic hormone) secretion in response to distension of the left atrium.[24] This mechanism may have partly accounted for the weight losses induced by spaceflight in all astronauts before the Skylab missions. The increased space available in Skylab (294 m³ (10 383 ft³))[3] permitted measurement of mass during flight (weight cannot be measured in the absence of gravity) using a spring mass oscillator.[25] This machine measures the period of oscillation of a mass set in linear oscillation between two springs; the period is related to mass and allows measurement to an accuracy of 0·01%. Daily measurements showed that the astronauts rapidly lost 1–2 kg (2·2–4·4 lb) within 3–4 days, which was probably due to fluid loss. This was followed by a slow but steady decline in mass during the rest of the flight attributable to loss of muscle and fat.[25]

In all Skylab crew members the net loss of fluid was caused by suppression of thirst rather than by diuresis. On average each astronaut excreted 400 ml less urine over the first 6 days of flight than over an equivalent period before flight, and water intake was decreased by an average of 900 ml.[26] Over the same period the urine osmolality also increased and was associated with increased urinary arginine vasopressin values early in flight. Twenty-four hour urinary excretion of sodium and potassium was increased throughout flight in most of the Skylab astronauts, and during this period all nine crew members had increased urinary aldosterone values, which could account for the urinary losses of potassium but not of sodium.[26] Increases in urinary aldosterone also occurred in the crew during the second half of the Apollo 17 mission, but a negative sodium balance persisted.[27]

The mechanism of increased sodium excretion remains unclear. In studies of human subjects immersed in water, natriuresis begins within the first hour and is accompanied by kaliuresis and diuresis[28] (but a true diuresis has never been documented during space flight). These changes are associated with depressed arginine vasopressin secretion and suppression of the renin–angiotensin-aldosterone system.[29,30] Injection of arginine vasopressin, although suppressing the diuresis, does not, however, prevent the natriuresis.[31] A natriuretic factor may be present in the urine of subjects immersed in water,[32] and a natriuretic hormone has been isolated,[33] so that the sodium loss during microgravity may depend on the increased secretion of such a substance.[10] Atrial natriuretic factor has indeed been shown to increase at first and then to decrease during shuttle flights.[34]

Whether central volumes and pressures are returned to normal preflight values by these homeostatic mechanisms is not known. The persistent facial puffiness suggests that they are not and raises the question of whether long term microgravity will induce changes in cardiac function comparable with those in patients with cardiac failure.

Recent evidence from the 1991 SLS-1 shuttle mission has led to a re-examination of the postulated mechanisms underlying the postflight fall in plasma volume described above.[35] During this flight, central venous pressure was shown to be normal or slightly lower than normal, rather than raised, in the single subject assessed: a finding in accord with earlier measurements of peripheral venous pressure. A new hypothesis suggests that the observed physiological changes are a consequence of certain physical changes associated with microgravity: a headward shift in abdominal contents, body elongation, and adoption of the fetal position all leading to an increase in the normal (0·133–0·4 kPa (1–3 mmHg)) transdiaphragmatic pressure gradient. The resulting *reduction* in atrial pressure leads to inferior vena caval and visceral engorgement (and especially of the liver and pancreas). Pancreatic involvement may explain the prediabetic pattern of glucose tolerance test seen after flight, and may therefore have implications for selection as astronauts of those believed to be prone to diabetes mellitus.

Respiratory function tests on the SLS-1 mission lend indirect support to the pressure change theory. Ventilation–perfusion gradients were shown to persist in microgravity: a phenomenon which can be explained if there is an increased pressure difference across the diaphragm produced by the cephalad movement of abdominal contents.

The new postulate does not explain some of the endocrine changes seen in microgravity, however, and specifically the mechanisms underlying the fall in arginine vasopressin levels. Non-human primate research has shown that such a fall can be induced by even a slight rise in cerebrospinal fluid pressure such as is seen in microgravity, in the absence of atrial distension. And other experimental work suggests that the Gauer–Henry reflex may not operate as originally believed.[35]

As with most research in microgravity, much additional work will be needed before these mechanisms are fully understood, but studies such as those on SLS-1 have demonstrated the ability of space medicine to contribute in ways impossible on earth to the clarification of fundamental physiological problems.

All astronauts have undergone electrocardiographic monitoring during flight, but no abnormalities were recorded until Apollo 15. The bigeminal beats and premature contractions (atrial and ventricular) which occurred during activity on the lunar surface and the return flight to earth were attributed to potassium deficit.[13,36] Potassium supplements did not, however, prevent similar potassium losses during the Apollo 17 mission, a flight in which no dysrhythmias were noted.[27] During Skylab missions, prolonged PR intervals were recorded in all astronauts and were attributed to increased vagal tone.[37] Sporadic ventricular ectopics also occurred but there was never any evidence to suggest myocardial ischaemia.[37] Extensive studies carried out on the Skylab astronauts after flight indicated that despite reductions in left ventricular end diastolic volume, stroke volume, and left ventricular mass no appreciable alteration in cardiac function had occurred.[38] Other indices of cardiovascular performance in microgravity confirm that, once hydrostatic realignment has occurred, behaviour is essentially normal. Thus, there is a slight increase in resting heart rate, but cardiac output and stroke volume are unchanged.[10]

The most important effect of the cephalad shift of fluid in microgravity is the temporary orthostatic intolerance that occurs when blood is pooled in the legs as a result of returning to normal gravity. This was demonstrated—for example, after the Apollo missions—by a fall in systolic pressure, a narrowing of pulse pressure, and an increased heart rate in response to lower body negative pressure.[39] These responses were exaggerated compared with preflight findings and were also associated with an increased incidence of presyncopal symptoms. Exercise tolerance was also reduced for up to 36 hours after flight.[40]

During the Skylab missions, determination of lower body negative pressure responses during flight indicated that orthostatic intolerance improved slightly after 30–50 days of microgravity but the tests remained more stressful than before flight.[41] Soviet studies of missions of up to 237 days have suggested that cardiovascular changes do not progress after 2–3 months in space.[10] More recently, the potentially serious effects of orthostasis were demonstrated by severe decompensation in a returning shuttle astronaut: even the seemingly mild re-entry acceleration of 1·2 Gz being sufficient in this case to cause syncope. Both American and Soviet astronauts now use anti-G trousers, inflated before re-entry, to reduce peripheral pooling of blood and consequent cardiovascular stress. However, this and other countermeasures, such as saline ingestion by cosmonauts, have not proved entirely effective and so the creation of artificial gravity may be the only complete solution to the problems of cardiovascular deconditioning in microgravity.

Musculoskeletal system

The force of gravity is probably the most enduring environmental feature of evolution on earth: it is responsible for determining the type and extent of physical skeletal support required by a species, for the manner of its circulatory supply and innervation, and for the appropriate disposition of musculature. Microgravity reduces the muscular effort required to perform physical tasks and to control posture, and so demands a readjustment of musculoskeletal organisation.

During the early phases of manned spaceflight programmes, because of the relatively short duration of the flights (for example, a maximum 302 hours in the Apollo series) muscle atrophy was not an important problem, although when investigated in Apollo 16 leg volume was found to be decreased.[13] And changes in gait, attributed to reduced muscle tone, were noted after flight in the crew of Soyuz 9, a Soviet mission lasting 425 hours.[20]

It was during the Skylab missions, when biostereometric analysis using stereophotogrammetry was used to measure the total and regional body volumes of the astronauts, that the true significance of the effects of microgravity on the musculoskeletal system was first appreciated. All but one of the nine crew lost muscle from the legs and probably also from other parts of the body such as the trunk.[42] Muscle atrophy was accompanied by increased urinary excretion of nitrogen (with an average rise of 4·0 g a day over preflight values) and phosphorus (a negative shift to 222–400 mg per day).[43] Muscle strength was also compared before and after flight using an isokinetic dynamometer. The different exercise regimens used on each mission showed that muscle exercising devices could reduce atrophy. Nevertheless, loss of strength from the arms was less than that from the legs, probably because everyday tasks in space require greater use of the arms,[44] a conclusion supported by the significant reduction in size of all muscles needed for standing and moving during the SLS-1 study. Overall, it has been estimated that during flight an exercise level of $80–100$ W min day^{-1} kg^{-1} body mass would be needed to prevent leg muscle atrophy.[42]

Undoubtedly, the single most important long term effect of microgravity is the inexorable demineralisation of bone, which is as yet unpreventable. During the Gemini flights X-ray densitometry showed reductions of 2–25% in the density of the astronauts' bones,[45] but the methods used were later found to be inaccurate. In later Apollo and all Skylab flights, the more sensitive technique of photon absorptiometry was used.[44] Area scans conducted on the Skylab crews indicated that no bone mineral was lost from the radius or the ulna on any of the three missions. Loss from the os calcis was not seen on the first (28-day) mission but a reduction of 7·4% was recorded in one astronaut on the second (59-day) flight. It was also found in two ($-4·5\%$ and $-7·9\%$) of the three crew members during the final (84-day) excursion.[46] Bone loss seems, therefore, to be regional with greater losses from trabecular than from cortical bone. In studies of rats exposed to prolonged microgravity trabecular bone volume was decreased and periosteal bone formation inhibited.[47]

The amount of bone lost by individual Skylab astronauts correlated with the severity of each man's negative calcium balance. This negative balance, which was seen in all the crew, was characterised by an increase in urinary calcium excretion beginning soon after entry into orbit and persisting throughout flight, and a progressive decrease in net intestinal absorption as shown by increased faecal calcium.[43] The urinary losses averaged about 4 g of calcium a month (or 0·3–0·4% of total body calcium), and continued until return to earth. By extrapolation, clinical osteoporosis may be predicted to occur after 4–8 months in space, with the consequent risk of fracture on return to normal gravity. Furthermore, although thin trabeculae can regain their normal thickness, trabeculae that have been lost completely cannot be restored. An understanding of the aetiology of bone loss and the development of prophylaxis or treatment will be vital to future extended space missions, although it is probable that the changes occurring during spaceflight affect bone structure (distribution) more than total bone mass.[48]

Bed rest and immobilisation produce a hypercalciuria similar to that seen in microgravity,[49] so that disuse is a probable aetiological factor, but the actual mechanisms are not yet known. Plasma samples obtained in flight showed increased parathyroid hormone concentrations in some (but not all) of the Skylab astronauts compared with preflight values.[26] Such increases were paradoxical in view of concomitant increases in plasma calcium concentrations. Because of the problems of measuring small changes in the concentrations of parathyroid hormone, its function in bone resorption in space must remain uncertain, although increased parathyroid hormone concentrations have been reported during immobility,[50] and in animals immobilisation osteoporosis is prevented by parathyroidectomy.[51]

Prevention of demineralisation by diet has not yet been systematically investigated during flight, but diet has been found to be ineffective in patients treated with bed rest. Furthermore, hormonal intervention—for example with calcitonin—has had no protective effect in such patients, although carefully controlled doses of diphosphonates, which inhibit bone resorption, may provide a remedy in the future.[52] The Skylab results also showed that demineralisation continued despite extensive exercise regimens, so that artificial gravity may again have to be provided either continuously by rotating the spacecraft or intermittently by small centrifuges within the cabin. The latter approach was successful in preventing decalcification in rats after 19.5 days aboard Cosmos 936 compared with an uncentrifuged control group.[53] Despite the continuing and intense research interest in this aspect of space physiology, evidence from cosmonauts undertaking long duration missions suggests that, at least when all known or potentially beneficial countermeasures are invoked, skeletal changes, although they occur with a severity directly related to the length of exposure, are not as profound as at first predicted.

Other changes

Although physiology and medicine have rarely been the principal topics of investigation during human spaceflight, a vast amount of data has been accumulated on many variables in addition to those described above.[54] The interpretation of most of these data is at best intelligently speculative and dedicated studies will be required before the mechanisms of change associated with microgravity can be fully elucidated. Nevertheless, fig 12.1 suggests some of the ways in which the changes seen may be interrelated. Some of the observations are worthy of additional comment.

● A reduction in the number of erythrocytes per unit volume and of haemoglobin concentration has been a consistent finding during and after flight in both the American and the Soviet programmes. It is now believed that the decline in plasma volume associated with microgravity leads to a relative increase in red cell mass and hence to inhibition of erythropoiesis. Inhibition is also

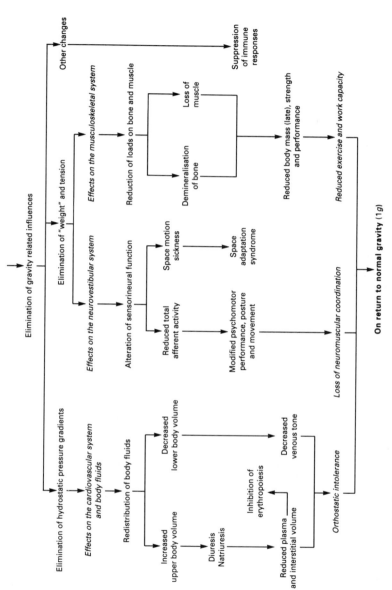

FIG 12.1.—Physiological consequences of exposure to microgravity.

205

triggered by the reduction in total oxygen requirement as a consequence of the reduced energy needs of the musculoskeletal and other systems.[10]

● Interestingly, the inflight measurement of a number of hormones concerned with the body's reaction to stress suggest that exposure to microgravity is not a prolonged stress stimulus: an increase in plasma cortisol and growth hormone, a reduction in adrenocorticotrophic hormone and insulin, and either a reduction or no change in catecholamines have been observed.[10] After flights of 8–11 months duration, however, plasma cortisol, growth hormone, insulin, thyroxine and catecholamines were all increased.

● Finally, long duration spaceflight produces unwelcome changes in both the humoral and cell-mediated immune systems, although the changes are not directly related to length of flight. Thus the reactivity of lymphocytes to phytohaemagglutinin (that is, their ability to synthesise nucleic acid) is diminished, the number of T lymphocytes in the blood falls, and T helper cells are less active. Furthermore, these attributes are suppressed until about 2–4 weeks after flight.[10] Such degradation of protection may increase the dangers of bacterial, viral or allergic disease, as well as potentiate autoimmune disorders.

Behavioural aspects

Human spaceflight was the almost exclusive preserve of military and civilian test pilots until the advent of the shuttle, with its crews of pilot astronauts, mission specialists, and payload specialists. The early astronaut and cosmonaut cadres comprised highly selected, highly motivated, and highly trained individuals for whom spaceflight alone was the goal. With the inevitable advance of manned spaceflight programmes, it is equally inevitable that future crews will include individuals with widely differing backgrounds and disciplines, with varying motivating drives, of different ethnic origins, and of both sexes. Greater attention must therefore be paid to the psychophysiological or behavioural aspects of spaceflight, including the problems of crew selection and training, isolation and confinement, sensory overload, group interactions, and circadian rhythms.[55] Furthermore, as flights become longer in duration and in absolute distance away from the earth, the problems of spacecraft habitability (such as architecture and design, ergonomics, sleep and leisure facilities, clothing and

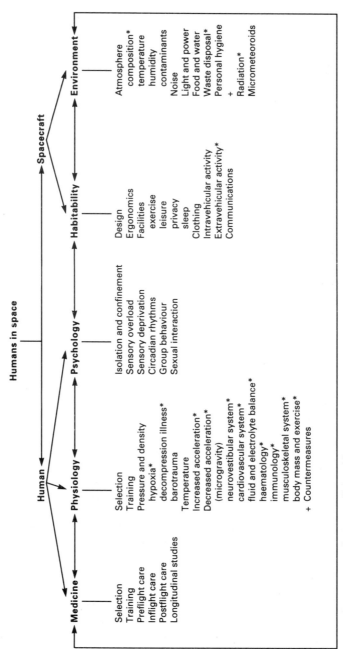

FIG 12.2—The scope of space medicine. *See text.

communication) will require further study and resolution,[3] as will the medical care and training for all phases of a mission:[56] fig 12.2 shows the complexity and extent of space medicine in its broadest sense.

1 Glaister DH. Physiological problems associated with acceleration in space flight. *J Br Interplan Soc* 1968; **21:** 154–65.
2 Berry CA. Summary of medical experience in the Apollo 7 through 11 manned spaceflights. *Aerospace Med* 1970; **41:** 500–19.
3 Harding RM. *Survival in space—the medical problems of manned spaceflight.* London: Routledge, 1989.
4 Glaister DH. Effect of accleration. In: West JB, ed. *Regional differences in the lung.* London: Academic Press, 1977: 323–79.
5 Alexander WC, Sever RJ, Hoppin FG. Hypoxemia induced in man by sustained forward accleration while breathing pure oxygen in a five pounds per square inch absolute environment. *Aerospace Med* 1966; **37:** 372–8.
6 Mandrovsky BN. Soyuz-9 flight, manned biomedical mission. *Aerospace Med* 1971; **42:** 172–7.
7 Denison DM, Howard P, Ernsting J, Cresswell AW. Fire risks in space capsules. *Nature* 1967; **213:** 648.
8 Mengel CE, Kann HE. Effects of in vivo hyperoxia on erythrocytes. III In vivo peroxidation of erythrocyte lipid. *J Clin Invest* 1966; **45:** 1150–8.
9 Johnson PC, Driscoll TB, LeBlanc AD. Blood volume changes. In: Johnson RS, Dietlein LF, eds. *Biomedical results from Skylab.* Washington: National Aeronautics and Space Administration, 1977: 235–41. (NASA SP-377.)
10 Grigoriev AI, Egorov AD. The effects of prolonged spaceflights on the human body. In: Bonting SL, ed. *Advances in space biology and medicine.* London: JAI Press, 1991, **1:** 1–35.
11 Jones WL. Individual life support systems outside a spacecraft cabin, space suits and capsules. In: Calvin M, Gazenko OG, eds. *Foundations of space biology and medicine. Vol 3. Space medicine and biotechnology.* Washington: National Aeronautics and Space Administration, 1975: 193–223.
12 Newell HE. The space environment. *Science* 1960; **131:** 385–90.
13 Berry CA. View of human problems to be addressed for long-duration space flight. *Aerospace Med* 1973; **44:** 1136–46.
14 Bailey VJ, Hoffman RA, English RA. Radiological protection and medical dosimetry for the Skylab crewmen. In: Johnston RS, Dietlein LF, eds. *Biomedical results from Skylab.* Washington: National Aeronautics and Space Administration, 1977: 64–9. (NASA SP-377).
15 Bjurstedt H. *Biology and medicine in space.* Paris: European Space Agency, 1979.
16 Graybiel A, Miller EF, Homick JL. Experiment M131. Human vestibular function. In: Johnston RS, Dietlein LF, eds. *Biomedical results from Skylab.* Washington: National Aeronautics and Space Administration, 1977: 74–103. (NASA SP-377.)
17 Davis JR, Vanderploeg JM, Santy PA, Jennings RT, Stewart DF. Space motion sickness during 24 flights of the space shuttle. *Aviat Space Environ Med* 1988; **59:** 1185–9.
18 Benson AJ. Possible mechanisms of motion and space sickness. In: Burke WR, Guyenne TD, eds. *Life-sciences research in space.* Paris: European Space Agency, 1977: 101–8. (ESA SP-130.)
19 Graybiel A. Space motion sickness: Skylab revisited. *Aviat Space Environ Med* 1980; **51:** 814–22.
20 Chekirda IF, Bogdashevskiy RB, Yeremin AV, Kolosov IA. Co-ordination structure of walking of Soyuz 9 crewmembers before and after flight. *Kosmichesk Biol Med (Moskva)* 1971; **5:** 71–7.
21 Arborelius M, Balldin UI, Lilja B, Lundgren CEG. Haemodynamic changes in man during immersion with the head above water. *Aerospace Med* 1972; **43:** 592–8.
22 Thornton WE, Hotter GW, Rummel JA. Anthropometric changes and fluid shifts. In: Johnston SR, Dietlein LF, eds. *Biomedical results from Skylab.* Washington: National Aeronautics and Space Administration 1977: 330–8. (NASA SP-377.)
23 Gibson EG. Skylab 4 crew observations. In: Johnston SR, Dietlein LF, eds. *Biomedical results from Skylab.* Washington: National Aeronautics and Space Administration 1977: 22–6. (NASA SP-377.)

24 Gauer OH, Henry JP. Neurohormonal control of plasma volume. In: Guyton AC, Cowley AW, eds. *International review of physiology. Cardiovascular physiology.* Vol. 9. Baltimore: University Park Press, 1976: 145–90.
25 Thornton WE, Ord J. Physiological mass measurements in Skylab. In: Johnston RS, Dietlein LF, eds. *Biomedical results from Skylab.* Washington: National Aeronautics and Space Administration, 1977: 175–82. (NASA SP-377.)
26 Leach CS, Rambaut PC. Biochemical responses of the Skylab crewmen: an overview. In: Johnston RS, Dietlein LF, eds. *Biomedical results from Skylab.* Washington: National Aeuronautics and Space Administration 1977: 204–16. (NASA SP-377.)
27 Leach CS, Rambaut PC, Johnston PC. Adrenocortical responses of the Apollo 17 crew members. *Aerospace Med* 1974; **45:** 529–34.
28 Epstein M, Duncan DC, Fishman LM. Characterization of the natriuresis caused in normal man by immersion in water. *Clin Sci* 1972; **43:** 275–87.
29 Epstein M, Pins DS, Miller M. Suppression of ADH during water immersion in normal man. *J Appl Physiol* 1975; **38:** 1038–44.
30 Epstein M, Saruta T. Effects of water immersion on renin–aldosterone and renal sodium handling in normal man. *J Appl Physiol* 1971; **31:** 368–74.
31 Khosla SS, Dubois AB. Fluid shifts during initial phase of immersion diuresis in man. *J Appl Physiol* 1979; **46:** 703–8.
32 Epstein M, Bricker NS, Bourgoignie JJ. Presence of a natriuretic factor in urine of normal men undergoing water immersion. *Kidney Int* 1978; **13:** 152–8.
33 De Wardener HE. The natriuretic hormone. *Q J Exp Physiol* 1982; **67:** 371–6.
34 Leach-Huntoon C, Johnson PC, Cintron NM. Haematology, immunology, endocrinology and biochemistry. In: Nicogossian AE, Leach-Huntoon C, Pool SL, eds. *Space physiology and medicine,* 2nd edn. Philadelphia: Lea and Febiger, 1989: 222–39.
35 Sandler H. Things may not be what they seem. *Aviat Space Environ Med* 1993; **64:** 247–8.
36 Douglas WR. Current status of space medicine. *Aviat Space Environ Med* 1978; **49:** 902–4.
37 Smith RF, Stanton K, Stoop D, Brown D, Janusz W, King P. Vectorcardiographic changes during extended space flight (MO93): observations at rest and during exercise. In: Johnston RS, Dietlein LF, eds. *Biomedical results from Skylab.* Washington: National Aeronautics and Space Administration, 1977: 339–49. (NASA SP-377.)
38 Henry WL, Epstein SE, Griffiths JM, Goldstein RE, Redwood DR. Effect of prolonged space flight on cardiac function and dimensions. In: Johnston RS, Dietlein LF, eds. *Biomedical results from Skylab.* Washington: National Aeronautics and Space Administration, 1977: 366–71. (NASA SP-377.)
39 Hoffer GW, Wolthuis RA, Johnson RL. Apollo space crew cardiovascular evaluations. *Aerospace Med* 1974; **45:** 807–20.
40 Rummel JA, Michel EL, Berry CA. Physiological response to exercise after space flight Apollo 7 to Apollo 11. *Aerospace Med* 1973; **44:** 235–8.
41 Johnson RL, Hoffer GW, Nicogossian AE, Bergman SA, Jackson MM. Lower body negative pressure: third manned Skylab mission. In: Johnston RS, Dietlein LF, eds. *Biomedical results from Skylab.* Washington: National Aeronautics and Space Administration, 1977: 284–312. (NASA SP-377.)
42 Whittle MW. Caloric and exercise requirements of space flight. I Biostereometric results from Skylab. *Aviat Space Environ Med* 1979; **50:** 163–7.
43 Whedon GD, Lutwak L, Rambaut PC *et al.* Mineral and nitrogen metabolic studies. In: Johnston RS, Dietlein LF, eds. *Biomedical results from Skylab.* Washington: National Aeronautics and Space Administration, 1977: 164–74. (NASA SP-377.)
44 Thornton EW, Rummel JA. Muscular deconditioning and its prevention in space flight. In: Johnston RS, Dietlein LF, eds. *Biomedical results from Skylab.* Washington: National Aeronautics and Space Administration, 1977: 191–7. (NASA SP-377.)
45 Mack PB, LaChance PA, Vose GP, Vogt FB. Bone demineralisation of foot and hand of Gemini–Titan IV, V and VI astronauts during orbital flight. *Am J Roentgenol Radium Ther Nucl Med* 1967; **100:** 503–11.
46 Smith MC, Rambaut PC, Vogel JM, Whittle MW. Bone mineral measurement experiment M078. In: Johnston RS, Dietlein LF, eds. *Biomedical results from Skylab.* Washington: National Aeronautics and Space Administration, 1977: 183–90. (NASA SP-377.)
47 Wronski TJ, Morey-Holton E, Jee WSS. Cosmos 1129: spaceflight and bone changes. *Physiologist* 1980; **23** (suppl.): S79–S82.
48 Morey-Holton ER, Arnaud SB. Skeletal responses to spaceflight. In: Bonting SL, ed. *Advances in space biology and medicine.* London: JAI Press, 1991; **1:** 37–69.

49 Hattner RS, McMillan DE. Influence of weightlessness upon the skeleton: a review. *Aerospace Med* 1968; **39:** 849–55.
50 Lerman S, Canterbury JM, Reiss E. Parathyroid hormone and the hypercalcaemia of immobilization. *J Clin Endocrinol Metab* 1977; **45:** 425–8.
51 Burckhardt JM, Jowsey J. Parathyroid and thyroid hormones in the development of immobilization osteoporosis. *Endocrinology* 1967; **81:** 1053–62.
52 Avioli L, Biglieri EG, Daughaday W, Raiaz LG, Reichlin S, Vogel J. Endocrinology. In: *Life beyond the earth's environment.* Washington: National Academy of Sciences, 1979: 45–66.
53 Kotovskaya AR, Ilyin EA, Korolkov VI, Shipov AA. Artificial gravity in space flight. *Physiologist* 1980; **23** (suppl.): S27–S28.
54 Nicogossian AE. Overall physiological response to space flight. In: Nicogossian AE, Leach-Huntoon C, Pool SL, eds. *Space physiology and medicine,* 2nd edn. Philadelphia: Lea and Febiger, 1989: 139–53.
55 Harding RM. Medical aspects of special types of flight—manned spacecraft. In: Ernsting J, King PF, eds. *Aviation medicine,* 2nd edn. London: Butterworths, 1988: 487–8.
56 Harding RM. Medical support for manned spaceflight. *Aviat Med Q* 1988; **2:** 43–55.

Index